The Health Professionals Guide to Delivering

Psychological Care for Men With Prostate Cancer

AF690671

Suzanne K Chambers AO, PhD
Nicole Heneka, PhD
Jeff Dunn AO, PhD

A *Facing the Tiger*
Psychological Care Resource

AUSTRALIANACADEMICPRESS

This guide has been developed to support health professionals in the delivery of psychological care for men with prostate cancer. It is designed to be used in conjunction with the book *Facing the Tiger: A Survivorship Guide for Men with Prostate Cancer and their Partners* published in 2020.

First published 2021 by Australian Academic Press Group Pty. Ltd.
Samford Valley, Australia www.australianacademicpress.com.au

Copyright © 2021 Suzanne K. Chambers, Nicole Heneka, Jeff Dunn

Copying for educational purposes
The *Australian Copyright Act 1968* (Cwlth) (Act) allows a maximum of one chapter or 10% of this book, whichever is the greater, to be reproduced and/or communicated by any educational institution for its educational purposes provided that the educational institution (or the body that administers it) has given a remuneration notice to Copyright Agency (CA) (www.copyright.com.au) under the Act.

For details of the CA licence for educational institutions contact:
Copyright Agency, Level 12, 66 Goulburn St. Sydney NSW 2000.
E-mail info@copyright.com.au

Production and communication for other purposes
Except for allowed content in this book defined as Page 4, Page 6, Appendix 2, Appendix 4 and Appendix 5 and usage defined as personal use by a health professional in the process of one-on-one therapy, and as permitted under the *Australian Copyright Act 1968* (Cwlth), for example a fair dealing for the purposes of study, research, criticism or review, no part of this book may be reproduced, stored in a retrieval system, or transmitted in any form or by any means electronic, mechanical, photocopying, recording or otherwise without prior written permission of the Copyright Holder. For all enquiries, contact the Publisher.

NATIONAL LIBRARY OF AUSTRALIA
A catalogue record for this book is available from the National Library of Australia

The Health Professionals Guide to Delivering Psychological Care for Men With Prostate Cancer
ISBN 9781925644555

DISCLAIMER: Every effort has been made in preparing this work to provide information based on accepted standards and practice at the time of publication. The publisher and authors, however, make no representations or warranties with respect to the accuracy or completeness of the contents of this book and specifically disclaim any implied warranties of merchantability or fitness for a particular purpose. It is sold on the understanding that the publisher is not engaged in rendering professional services and neither the publisher nor the authors shall be liable for damages arising herefrom. If professional advice or other expert assistance is required, the services of a competent professional should be sought.

Publisher & Editor: Stephen May
Cover design: Luke Harris, Working Type Studio
Typesetting: Australian Academic Press
Printing: Lightning Source

"The good physician knows his patients through and through, and his knowledge is bought dearly. Time, sympathy and understanding must be lavishly dispensed, but the reward is to be found in that personal bond which forms the greatest satisfaction of the practice of medicine. One of the essential qualities of the clinician is interest in humanity, for the secret of the care of the patient is in caring for the patient."

F.W. Peabody. The care of the patient JAMA Vol. 88, pp. 877-882, Mar. 19, 1927

Dedicated to our friend and colleague Dr Jimmie Holland (1928–2017) and her favourite quote.

Acknowledgements

Tennessee Williams once said that time is the longest distance between two places, and nowhere is that more evident than in the changed landscape of prostate cancer survivorship since the original publication of *Facing the Tiger: A Survivorship Guide for Men with Prostate Cancer and their Partners* in 2013.

Once distant and disconnected voices have come together, and we find ourselves facing a new horizon for prostate cancer care.

We wish to thank those who contributed their time and expertise in helping us bring this manual to life — Dr Chris Nelson from the Memorial Sloane Kettering Cancer Centre, Queensland-based clinical psychologist Samantha Clutton, Professors Daniel Galvao and Robert Newton from Edith Cowan University, Professor Mark Lazenby from the University of California Irvine, Professor John Oliffe from the University of British Columbia, Clinical Sexologist Melissa Hadley Barrett, and Adjunct Professor Sally Sara and her esteemed colleague (Captain) Bernie Riley from Prostate Cancer Foundation of Australia, and along with them the indefatigable Anne Savage.

Equally, we wish to acknowledge our profound gratitude to the passionate clinicians, nurses, and allied health workers who serve as part of the national and international urological community, inspiring our progress through their everyday actions.

Finally, we offer our deepest thanks to the thousands of men and their families facing prostate cancer, who have shown us that the greatest change occurs when we care.

We tip our hats to you, the reader, for making the commitment to use this guide as your compass.

Suzanne Chambers, Nicole Heneka, Jeff Dunn
December 2021

Contents

Chapter 3

The Foundation Components of a Facing the Tiger Intervention

Chapter 4

Flexible Component 1: Psychoeducation — Coping with a Prostate Cancer Diagnosis

Chapter 5

Flexible Component 2: Stress Management and Wellbeing

Chapter 6

Flexible Component 3: Treatment Decision Making

Chapter 7

Flexible Component 4: Managing Relationships Under Stress

Chapter 8

Flexible Component 5: Problem solving

Chapter 9

Flexible Component 6: Managing Difficult Thoughts

Chapter 10

Flexible Component 7: Pivoting to Valued Directions

Chapter 11

Flexible Component 8: Masculinity and Prostate Cancer

Chapter 12

Flexible Component 9: Prostate Cancer and Sexual Relationships

Appendix 2: Client Handouts

Professor Suzanne K Chambers AO, PhD

Professor Suzanne Chambers AO is a health psychologist and registered nurse who has been working as a practitioner-researcher in psycho-oncology for over 30 years. She was awarded her PhD in 2004 within the School of Psychology at Griffith University and has over 300 peer-reviewed publications and numerous books, book chapters and monographs. Her work has focussed on developing models to predict help-seeking and adjustment after cancer: designing remote access psychological interventions for people affected by cancer, integrating peer support into controlled design methodologies, and integrating distress screening into interventions to target high distress cancer patient groups. Professor Chambers was appointed an Officer in the General Division of the Order of Australia (AO) in 2018 for distinguished service to medical research, particularly in the area of psycho-oncology and to community health through patient care strategies to assist men with prostate cancer. She is a Board member of Healthy Male (Andrology Australia) and an Honorary Fellow with St Vincent's Health Network Sydney. Professor Chambers is Executive Dean of the Faculty of Health Sciences at the Australian Catholic University.

Dr Nicole Heneka, PhD

Dr Nicole Heneka is a Postdoctoral Research Fellow with the National Health and Medical Research Council Centre for Research Excellence in Prostate Cancer Survivorship at the University of Technology Sydney. She has over 20 years experience in program management and has focussed on health services research in cancer and palliative care services for the last 12 years. In her current role, she leads a program of research in the delivery of prostate cancer survivorship care, including patterns of care, implementation and evaluation strategies for survivorship care, and research capacity building in survivorship care. Dr Heneka's work in health services research has been recognised through her award of the Clinical Excellence Commission Ian O'Rourke Scholarship in Patient Safety (2016), and the Palliative Care Australia, National Emerging Researcher award (2019).

Professor Jeff Dunn AO, PhD

Professor Jeff Dunn AO is the Chief of Mission and Head of Research at the Prostate Cancer Foundation of Australia and President-Elect of the Union for

International Cancer Control (UICC). His work in cancer control spans 30 years, during which time he has dedicated his career to the development of strategies that underpin cancer survival and improve awareness of the disease. He is a recognised World Cancer Leader and, prior to his appointment as UICC President-Elect, served as Treasurer of the UICC for four years and as an Elected Director for six. Professor Dunn also serves as the Professor and Chair of Social and Behavioural Science at the University of Southern Queensland, where his work has a central focus on the social and behavioural aspects of cancer, covering the continuum of research, prevention, early detection, supportive care, and quality of life. He is actively involved in research in this field and is also a Director of the West Moreton Hospital and Health Service Board and Chair of the Risk and Audit Committee. He was appointed as an Officer in the Order of Australia (2014) for distinguished service to medical administration through leadership of cancer control organisations and promotion of innovative and integrated cancer care programs.

Chapter 1

Understanding the Facing the Tiger Psychological Care Approach

Why 'Facing the Tiger'?

Being diagnosed with cancer is a frightening experience for most people, a threat to life and the future, not unlike being faced with a fearful and imminent danger — like facing a tiger. Prostate cancer is no exception. Men who are diagnosed with prostate cancer are at risk of heightened psychological distress,[1-3] often have high unmet psychological support needs,[4-6] and have a 70% greater risk of suicide than men in the general population.[7]

Almost one-third of men with prostate cancer will experience some form of psychological distress across both the treatment spectrum and different stages of the disease.[1,3] Compared with men in the general population, men with prostate cancer are twice as likely to experience depression and three times more likely to experience anxiety.[8] The risk of suicide for these men is greatest within the first year after diagnosis,[7,9] and increases with the severity of the clinical stage of the disease at diagnosis.[10-12]

Prostate cancer treatment itself contributes to psychological distress, largely due to side effects that can be lifelong. Surgical and radiotherapy treatments, for example, may negatively affect sexual, urinary, and bowel functioning, which increases psychological distress.[13] Men undergoing androgen deprivation therapy (ADT) for prostate cancer experience poorer psychosocial outcomes than men receiving other treatments, including depression, anxiety, relationship changes, cognitive and affective symptoms, and sleep disturbances.[14-17] Regardless of other treatments, receiving ADT is predictive of higher distress,[17] and has a threefold greater risk of depression compared to radiation treatment alone.[18]

While research has regularly shown elevated levels of distress in men with prostate cancer, supportive care within the medical system for such distress remains poor. Unmet supportive care needs remain highly prevalent, particularly at the start of treatment when side effects are new or unknown and quality of life is first impacted[19]. Over 80% of men report unmet supportive care needs relating to sexual issues, psychological issues, health system and information issues in the first year after a prostate cancer diagnosis.[6] At 15-years post-diagnosis, over one-third of these men still report unmet physical, psychological, sexual, existential and informational needs.[17,19]

This unaddressed psychological distress in men with prostate cancer can result in poorer quality of life and clinical outcomes. [6,19,20] Yet, again, ameliorating such distress to improve outcomes is not yet a standard part of medical treatment for prostate cancer. Psychological interventions for men with prostate cancer are effective in reducing decision-related stress, depression and anxiety, improving mental health, domain-specific, and health-related quality of life.[21] There is clear evidence that a focus on psychological care improves **prostate cancer survivorship** outcomes.[20-22] However, despite routine clinical follow-up, many men with prostate cancer do not receive psychological interventions in a timely manner, if at all.

The purpose of the Facing the Tiger psychological care approach is to help health professionals provide accessible **low-intensity psychological care** early and at a time when it is most needed. The approach makes use of the book *Facing the Tiger: A Survivorship Guide for Men with Prostate Cancer and their Partners* (*Facing the Tiger*), an evidence-informed self-management resource. A complete copy of the book is reproduced for reference in this Guide in Appendix 6. The first edition of *Facing the Tiger* was released in 2013 in response to requests by men for a book focusing on the day-to-day worries and concerns they and their partners experience. It was updated in 2020 and incorporates the latest knowledge base in prostate cancer survivorship. Using the Facing the Tiger psychological care approach ensures the man is connected to a system of care that responds to his needs, can be tailored to his concerns, and can be escalated to other care systems when indicated. This contributes to better prostate cancer survivorship outcomes.

Prostate Cancer Survivorship

Cancer survivorship care supports wellbeing and quality of life across the cancer trajectory. There are numerous definitions and categories of survivorship that have evolved over time.[23-25] The definition used in the Facing the Tiger psychological care approach follows the National Institutes for Health, National Cancer Institute definition[26]:

> In cancer, survivorship focuses on the health and wellbeing of a person with cancer from the time of diagnosis until the end of life. This includes the physical, mental, emotional, social, and financial effects of cancer that begin at diagnosis and continue through treatment and beyond. The survivorship experience also includes issues related to follow-up care (including regular health and wellness check-ups), late effects of treatment, cancer recurrence, second cancers, and quality of life. Family members, friends, and caregivers are also considered part of the survivorship experience.
>
> An individual is considered a cancer survivor from the time of diagnosis and throughout the balance of their life. There are many types of survivors, including those living with cancer and those free of cancer. This term is meant to capture a population of those with a history of cancer rather than to provide a label that may or may not resonate with individuals.

Despite existing survivorship guidelines,[27,28] men with prostate cancer describe the prostate cancer survivorship experience as challenging, medically focused, and uncoordinated, resulting in unmet supportive care needs, distress and anxiety.[29] This has prompted calls for better coordinated and men-centred care that responds and articulates with masculine ways of being.[30]

To address these gaps, in 2020, a specialist 47-member panel was convened comprising leaders from key Australian and New Zealand clinical and community groups and consumers from diverse backgrounds, including LGBTQIA (Lesbian, Gay, Bisexual, Transgender, Queer and/or Questioning, Intersex, and Asexual and/or Ally), regional, rural and urban settings. Using surveys and meetings, the panel developed descriptors for men's current prostate cancer survivorship experience, along with survivorship elements that were assessed for importance and feasibility. From these, they defined six key domains of survivorship care that directly influence long-term physical and mental wellbeing,[30] and are focused on patient, versus process, outcomes:

- **Personal Agency:** patients are self-aware in assessing their needs, seeking assistance when required, and building resilience to manage their own health where possible.
- **Health Promotion and Advocacy:** increasing the community's knowledge of men's health and prostate cancer and supporting awareness and advocacy through the provision of up-to-date information.

- **Shared Management:** patients and health professionals work together to improve outcomes and ensure quality survivorship care with shared and informed decision making about all aspects of care.
- **Vigilance:** attentive surveillance of physical and psychosocial effects, comorbidities, recurrence and second cancers across the survivorship continuum from diagnosis to end-of-life care; this includes psychosocial effects on partners and family members.
- **Care Coordination:** men-centred care where patients and families arrive at the right place at the right time for the right care once a diagnosis has been made.
- **Evidence-based Survivorship Interventions:** providing accessible psychosocial and psychosexual care, exercise and physical activity, nutrition, peer support, financial assistance, and specialist nursing interventions.

The resulting *Prostate Cancer Survivorship Essentials Framework*[30] (Figure 1), has been widely endorsed by key cancer and urological groups. It is designed to guide the provision of integrated quality prostate cancer survivorship care in a

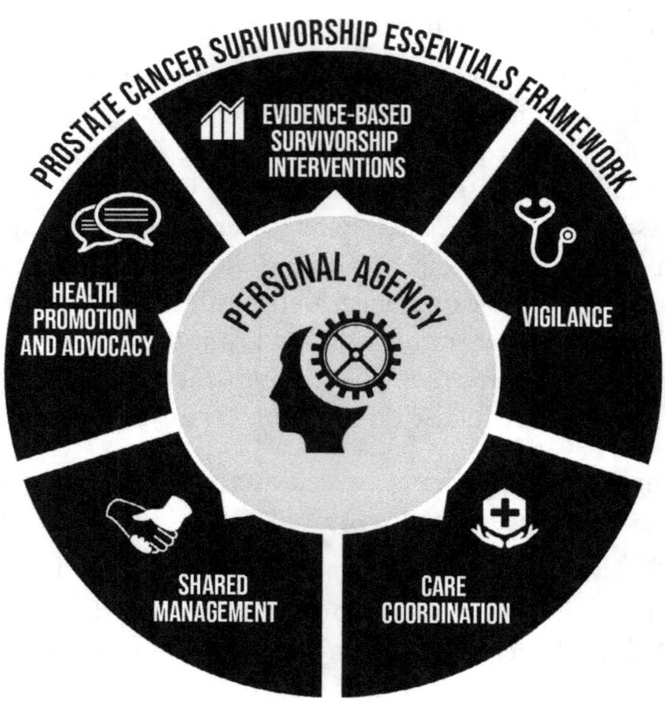

Figure 1: Prostate Cancer Survivorship Essentials Framework[30]

variety of settings. Importantly, the central domain relates to personal agency of a survivor as a key element that links all others, placing the man and his family at the centre of care.

Low-Intensity Psychological Care

Low-intensity interventions aim to democratise psychological care. Care that is widely accessible and designed to enhance personal agency encourages the person receiving care to become an agent in managing their personal experience in a way that encourages mastery of their wellbeing.

In a sense, this means the role of the health professional is to form a partnership with the patient and deliver care that includes coaching the man in understanding their experience of suffering, learning the skills to manage the challenges they may experience, and developing personal agency in how they choose to face the present and the future. In this partnership, each person — the health professional (who may come from a variety of backgrounds and experiences) and the patient (who also will come from a variety of backgrounds and experiences) — contributes knowledge and learning.

There are many expressions of low-intensity care.[31] Typically, this approach will:

- Match the intensity and focus of care to the level and type of need.
- Be person-centred where the context, values and priorities of the individual guide the intervention.
- Be evidence-informed.
- Connect to self-help that is client-paced.
- Link to community resources.

Matching Care to Need

After a prostate cancer diagnosis, the needs of men and their families vary greatly. These needs are influenced by life course, context and gender, and will change over time. Critically, care must be individualised to the level of need and be accessible in a range of settings, spanning community and acute care settings. Regular and routine distress screening is essential to match care to need and facilitates delivery of targeted care.[32]

A **tiered model of care**[33] (Figure 2) articulates between need, distress, and depth of care, over four levels. As needs increase, the depth of care increases and the intervention focus narrows and becomes more specialised.[33] This

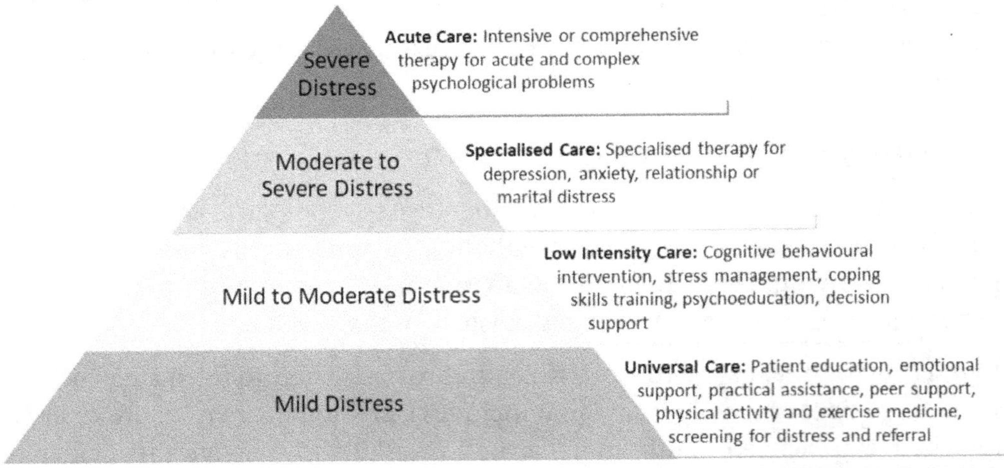

Figure 2. The Tiered Model of Psychosocial Care after Prostate Cancer
Adapted from the Tiered Model of Care[33]

framework is a guide with the understanding that care should be individualised to the preferences and context of the individual and their unique situation.

- **Universal Care:** This is psychosocial care that should be offered and available to all men with prostate cancer across their cancer experience. This level of care lays a foundation for more in-depth levels of intervention for men with higher needs or distress. Universal care includes informational support through patient health education, empathic emotional support, advice for practical concerns, peer support, physical activity, and screening for distress and referral.
- **Low-Intensity Care:** This care level provides additional support for men experiencing mild to moderate distress and/or who express a need for further support. It targets the challenges associated with a prostate cancer diagnosis in more depth. It includes psycho-education, stress and worry management, coping skills training including problem solving and goal setting, decision support, and communication strategies to enhance support networks. The *Facing the Tiger* book is an example of a low-intensity psychosocial care intervention.
- **Specialised Care:** This level of care is stepped-up for men who are experiencing moderate to severe distress that may be persistent and/or who express a need for additional support beyond what is

already provided. The intervention is individualised with a treatment plan targeting specific factors contributing to that individual's distress.

- **Acute Care:** This provides high level multi-disciplinary mental health care for men with severe distress and complex problems. These men may present with depression, anxiety or trauma symptoms that seriously impact their ability to function day-to-day. Since suicidal ideation may be present, these men require an immediate assessment and intervention with an initial focus on the assessment of safety and management of the acute crisis.

Being Person-Centred

Being person-centred means tailoring care to match the perspectives and needs of the person as an individual. First, this means understanding and responding to the life course and stage of life of the person you are caring for. This includes their age, family and partner situation, sexuality, cultural background, faith, lifestyle, and social and economic background, including health literacy.

It also means being responsive to masculine values (that will vary across life course) and delivering men-centred care responsive to these values. Men-centred care is contextual and dynamic and considers how health care services for men intersect with masculinity and with their preferences for prostate cancer care.

Evidence-informed

Multi-modal psychosocial and psychosexual interventions based on a firm research base effectively reduce psychological distress and improve survivorship outcomes for men with prostate cancer.[20-22] Effective interventions include combinations of psycho-education, cognitive-behavioural approaches, decision support, relaxation training, communication skills training, tailored supportive care, and peer support.[20-22]

Client-paced self-help

A flexible service delivery approach that emphasises elements of self-help encourages the man to choose the specific areas of concern he would like to work on and to manage personal change at a rate that is comfortable for him within his environment or context. Moving too fast or too slow runs the risk of the man disengaging from the process. A collaborative approach to care design will help tailor support to the pace that will work for each individual man. Many services will have specific guidelines around the duration and scheduling of psychological care services, some derived from available resources and some based on the experience and preferences of the service provider and their clinical approach to care. Being client-paced means bringing the man's preferences in as part of this consideration and supports the notion of patient autonomy.[34]

Community Resources

The earliest advocates for psychological support in cancer have been patients themselves who saw the gaps in care and stepped up to offer social support systems to address emotional, informational and tangible concerns.[35] Emotional support means feeling understood and able to share feelings and experiences. Informational support is having salient and helpful information about the problem being faced. Tangible support encompasses practical needs that relate to physical wellbeing. Having access to such types of social support can buffer a person from stressful events and also act as a coping resource.[36-38]

Across the globe, numerous community-led groups have been formed to support men with prostate cancer. These groups offer connections to peer support programs as well as educational and outreach programs. Several of these are listed at the end of this manual (Appendix 1). Health professionals working in support of men with prostate cancer should be aware of such local services and resources, their appropriateness, and their level of accessibility. Good psychological care includes awareness of the community resources available so that men can reach out to these if or when they feel these supports match their needs.

The Facing the Tiger Approach to Psychological Care and Survivorship

The Facing the Tiger psychological care approach to men with prostate cancer provides guidance on vigilance and surveillance of psychological wellbeing by incorporating screening for distress into regular care. The strategies used are informed by firm evidence, and the approach allows for a highly accessible, cost-effective, low-intensity psychological intervention centred on increasing a man's personal agency. By taking a holistic approach to psychological wellbeing that includes physical wellbeing, the principles of health promotion are integrated into survivorship care.

The approach is men-centred and strengths-based, using cognitive behavioural practice drawn from three main perspectives: **stress and coping**, **problem-solving**, and **psychological flexibility**. The linking element to these perspectives is that how a person thinks about their cancer and their situation or context, the way they respond to their thinking, and the consequent actions they take all interact to influence their psychological outcome. Specifically, the approach incorporates an understanding and responsiveness to masculine values in the design of care and in the identification of a man's personal strengths on which he can build his resilience in the face of the cancer diagnosis.

Stress and coping

The transactional theory of stress and coping was initially developed by Lazarus and Folkman,[39] and later revised by Folkman.[40,41] This theory is based on the dynamic cycles of thoughts and actions that people use to cope in stressful situations. People constantly appraise current or impending events in their environments. Events can be appraised either as positive or as challenging (leading to positive responses) or instead as threatening. If the latter, the resulting distress initiates coping strategies to manage the consequent emotions (*emotion-focused coping*) or to address the stressor itself (*problem-focused coping*). The process of coping changes the relationship between the person and their environment to produce an outcome that is reappraised by the person as favourable, unfavourable or unresolved. A favourable outcome produces positive emotions. But unfavourable or unresolved outcomes trigger further distress which either elicits negative emotions or triggers *meaning-focussed coping*, which draws on the individual's values, beliefs and goals to reorder priorities, relieve distress and sustain coping efforts over time.[41] Consequently, stress is a continuous process of appraisal, coping strategies and reappraisal which can elicit positive or negative emotions.[42]

Problem-solving

Men who have been diagnosed with prostate cancer may face a number of challenges or problems to manage, for example, urinary incontinence, sexual dysfunction, fatigue or loss of vitality, sarcopenia or other metabolic changes.[43] These problems can be long term and multilayered, and a cause for distress, social isolation and withdrawal. To meet these needs, the Facing the Tiger psychological care approach draws on the approach developed by Nezu and colleagues,[44] which applies a problem-solving approach to coping with cancer. Here the man is encouraged to define and formulate the problem, set goals for change, generate alternative actions or strategies to apply, evaluate possible outcomes for each strategy and from this, define a solution. The outcomes of the solution are then self-monitored and adapted as needed.

Psychological flexibility

Psychological flexibility as defined in the work of Steven Hayes[45] is based on the proposal that attending to the present moment and reflecting on uncomfortable thoughts and feelings in a non-judgemental, kind and curious way can provide the opportunity to uncover important yearnings and personal values. From this self-understanding, a person can pivot to personally valued goals and generate alternative ways of being or acting that are more likely to allow for movement and growth. Such flexibility provides an approach for change when a person feels 'stuck'.

Applying these perspectives together, a diagnosis of prostate cancer can be viewed as major life stress that is interpreted by the man as a threat — to his survival, to his sense of self, his lifestyle, and to his relationships. The unpleasant thoughts, feelings, and bodily sensations that occur in response to this threat interact to shape the man's lived experience of cancer. The context, being diagnosed with prostate cancer, is the environment that triggers the man's stress/distress response. With an understanding of his own response and this interaction, the man can potentially target each of these areas of focus to enhance his mastery of the situation and improve his mental wellbeing.

Using the *Facing the Tiger* Book

The *Facing the Tiger* book (*Facing the Tiger: A Survivorship Guide for Men with Prostate Cancer and their Partners)* plays a major role in the Facing the Tiger psychological care approach and is endorsed by the Prostate Cancer Foundation of Australia, Urological Society of Australia and New Zealand, and the Australia and New Zealand Urological Nurses Society, as well as recommended by experts worldwide and used by thousands of men and those who care for them. It intersects with the survivorship domains of vigilance, evidence-based interventions, personal agency, and health promotion and advocacy.

In practical terms, the book is designed so that each chapter focuses on a different challenge or problem, allowing men to direct their attention to what is most salient to them in the present moment. Each chapter includes authentic personal stories that mirror the therapeutic content of the chapter to normalise the issue and create a sense of a community of experience. As far as possible, the personal stories represent a diversity of experiences aiming to be inclusive.

Reflective exercises and activities are suggested in each chapter as 'homework' to aid learning and integration of the content into experience. For the health professional, this then allows them to use the relevant chapter as between-session homework that can be reviewed at the commencement of each subsequent contact.

Building a Facing the Tiger Intervention

Effective psychological intervention requires a trusting, non-judgemental and compassionate relationship between the health professional and the client. Before using any of the information and materials provided in this guide to run a Facing the Tiger psychological care intervention, it is important to understand the importance of establishing a therapeutic alliance.

Establishing a Therapeutic Alliance

For the health professional, this means being able to adopt the perspective of the man seeking help and seeing his situation through his eyes — to understand his view of where he is now, what matters most to him, and the life experiences that underpin this. In this level playing field, the man is the expert about his own experience. The health professional brings their expertise to work jointly with the man on the concerns that are most important to him.

There are three key elements to a successful therapeutic alliance: the bond between the man and the health professional (including trust, caring and respect), mutual agreement about the goals of the intervention (e.g., decreasing feelings of distress about prostate cancer), and agreement as to the way this will be approached (e.g., assessment of distress and wellbeing at regular intervals, systematically working through agreed problems, reviewing self-help materials).[46,47]

The task for the health professional is to assist the man to feel respected and safe to disclose problems and explore alternative coping options. Key to this process is effective rapport building which, once established, creates an environment in which individuals are motivated to develop their own solutions and experiment with new ideas. A strong and positive rapport can create safety to explore negative emotions and thoughts and encourage a sense of control and the development of the man's own resources. Health professionals who work to build trust, offer encouragement and generate a sense of ease with men are on the way to building rapport through emotional connectedness.

Begin by establishing the nature of the relationship and discussing the content and process of how you will work together each session. Throughout the process, men can be encouraged through recognition and acknowledgement of their strengths, resources, competencies and past achievements. Changes that display mastery of new self-management strategies can also be acknowledged. Examples of these could include completing or partially completing homework tasks, managing to solve a problem in dealing with a treatment side effect, or challenging or not reacting strongly to difficult thoughts.

Strategies to encourage a strong therapeutic alliance include asking for and being open to feedback, having an awareness of one's own limitations, and the opportunity for self-learning that presents with each session.

The extent to which a person with cancer feels supported is a major factor in improving psychological adjustment to their diagnosis and treatment.[48] Research indicates that good rapport building is predictive of positive supportive care outcomes, aids decision making, improves treatment satisfaction and encourages treatment and research compliance.[49] Further, a recent systematic review noted that a positive therapeutic alliance is in itself likely a driver of therapeutic change across a broad range of patients, clinical problems, and settings.[50] Hence establishing a strong alliance early and then maintaining this is critical to effective psychological care.

Building Intervention Sessions

A Facing the Tiger intervention is designed to be highly flexible so that support can be tailored to the man's needs and situation. Therefore, the health professional has the option to build the number and topic of sessions that best fits the needs of their client. Each session will include the two **Foundation Components** and at least one selected **Flexible Component** followed by **Homework**. Both foundation components are undertaken at the start of every session to help identify which flexible component is most appropriate for use in that session, and to identify if care needs to be escalated.

Each man with whom you are conducting sessions will require a copy of the self-management book *Facing the Tiger: A Survivorship Guide for Men with Prostate Cancer and their Partners*. The book is available both from the publisher's webstore (www.aapbooks.com) as well as most major online bookstores and on order from local bookstores. Suggested readings and activities from *Facing the Tiger* are included with each session component. A complete copy of *Facing the Tiger* is reproduced for reference in the back of this guidebook in Appendix 6.

At the end of each intervention session, outline the related homework and encourage the man to complete it before his next session. This helps to reinforce session content and support reflective learning.

While the inclusion of flexible components is tailored to the man's needs and situation, it is not necessary that every man be given sessions covering all the flexible components. It is strongly recommended though, that all men receive Flexible Component 1 (Psychoeducation) and Flexible Component 10 (Survivorship Care) timed to fit the man's priorities.

Foundation Components

Foundation One: Distress screening

The man's level of distress is assessed at the start of every session using the *Prostate Cancer Distress Screen*,[51] an ultra-short screening tool (See Appendix 3 for free download link). If the man scores at or above the cut-off point of 4, he should be further assessed for the presence of anxiety and/or depression. His care should then be focussed as appropriate (refer Foundation One page 17).

Foundation Two: Agenda setting

It is essential to establish clarity early on in the session about the man's agreed priorities and the key intervention components that are important for the man's experience now and as it evolves. This means that ***before delivering any session content***, the health professional should invite the man to talk about his current situation and what his main worries or concerns are. The *Problem Checklist* (see Appendix 3 for free download link) on which men are encouraged to note down any current problems or concerns can be used to generate session priorities. However, be aware that sometimes the key concern or problem might not emerge until after the session has advanced and rapport has been established. The health professional needs to be flexible to pivot to the man's stated concerns as they emerge but can circle back to initial expressed issues towards the end of the session.

Flexible Components

There are ten flexible components of a Facing the Tiger intervention, each of which is linked to a section of *Facing the Tiger*. It is intended that these linked chapters be used as a self-management resource for the man after each session.

- **Flexible Component 1:** Psychoeducation — Coping with a Prostate Cancer Diagnosis (Chapters 1 & 2)
- **Flexible Component 2**: Stress Management and Wellbeing (Chapter 8)
- **Flexible Component 3**: Treatment Decision Making (Chapter 5)
- **Flexible Component 4**: Managing Relationships Under Stress (Chapters 3 and 4)
- **Flexible Component 5**: Problem Solving (Chapter 9)
- **Flexible Component 6**: Managing Difficult Thoughts (Chapter 7)
- **Flexible Component 7**: Pivoting to Valued Directions (Chapters 10 & 11)
- **Flexible Component 8**: Masculinity and Prostate Cancer (Chapters 2, 6, 11)
- **Flexible Component 9**: Prostate Cancer and Sexual Relationships (Chapter 6)
- **Flexible Component 10:** Survivorship Care (Chapter 12)

Homework

A fundamental aspect of a Facing the Tiger intervention is that each man takes responsibility for working towards personal changes that will be beneficial for them and have a positive impact on their lives. In order to maximise the chance that the man will continue the self-work change he has covered in each session, it is best that he complete homework or practice between sessions.

Men are encouraged to identify their priorities for attention at the beginning of each session. At the end of each session, you should discuss with the man the agreed strategies that he will test out following the session and clarify any homework tasks. This way, the end of the session becomes a brief recap of what has been discussed and what might happen next.

Suggested readings and activities for homework from the *Facing the Tiger* book are included with each session component. *Facing the Tiger* also contains personal stories from other survivors that can help the man reflect more deeply on his own experience and give him new ideas about managing difficulties as they arise.

Component Structure

Each flexible component in this manual is set out in a standardised structure so you can easily build a program of intervention sessions and navigate the delivery. Each component includes:

- **Introduction:** An overview of the component for the health professional
- **Key Points**: Discussion points to include in the session.
- **Key Procedures**: A how-to guide for in-session activities (e.g., decision making) where applicable.
- **Homework**: Suggested readings and activities from *Facing the Tiger*.
- **Assessment**: Options for within-session assessment, including the Prostate Cancer Distress Screen.
- **Key Resources**: Overview of the related chapter in *Facing the Tiger*, as well as **activities** and **personal stories**.
- **Additional Resources**: Additional readings/resources/activities where applicable. Also, if applicable, this section will outline other related Flexible Components that may be useful for issues covered in the session.

  Specific weblinks to some resources are provided in the text with a scanable QR Code beside them so you can immediately go to the relevant website.

The Foundation Components of a Facing the Tiger Intervention

Foundation Component One: Distress Screening

Routine and regular screening for psychological distress is a core component of good cancer care.[52,53] Distress screening facilitates the rapid identification of patients who require additional in-depth psychological intervention. The Facing the Tiger psychological care approach uses a simple tool to assist health professionals when working with men with prostate cancer. The *Prostate Cancer Distress Screen* ('Distress Screen') consists of a single item Distress Scale and an accompanying Problem Checklist to help men and health care providers identify the drivers of distress and determine which type of intervention is indicated for the key challenges being faced. A link to a free downloadable PDF copy of the Distress Screen provided by the Prostate Cancer Foundation of Australia is included in Appendix 3.

The Distress Scale portion of the Distress Screen is an ultra-short screening tool that can be used to determine current distress levels and can be followed with more in-depth screening if needed.[54] It is a visual scale that is brief and simple to administer and score, making it ideal for use in any practice setting.[55] The Distress Scale asks patients how distressed they feel on an eleven-point scale, ranging from 0 (no distress) to 10 (extreme distress). This scale is well validated worldwide,[56-64] including in prostate cancer populations.[51]

Patients who report a distress score of 4 or greater should be further screened for depression, anxiety and suicidal ideation using tools such as those following.

Patient Health Questionnaire (PHQ-9)

This is used to monitor the severity of depression and response to treatment and can be used to make a tentative diagnosis of depression in at-risk populations. The scale includes an item for suicidal ideation (Item 9).[65] A photocopiable copy of this questionnaire along with a link to a free downloadable PDF copy is included in Appendix 5. Scoring instructions are available from https://www.phqscreeners.com.

Generalised Anxiety Disorder Assessment (GAD-7)

This is a well-validated screening tool and severity measure for generalised anxiety.[66] A photocopiable copy of this questionnaire along with a link to a free downloadable PDF copy is included in Appendix 5. Scoring instructions are available from https://www.phqscreeners.com.

Both of these tools are free to use and easy to complete. However, the choice of further screening tools is at the discretion of the health professional, and there are many validated tools to choose from.

Administering the Prostate Cancer Distress Screen

The Prostate Cancer Distress Screen is administered at the beginning of each session to assess distress levels and identify factors that may be contributing to the man's distress.

Assessments are conducted as follows.

- Introduce the rationale for distress screening within each session. Asking this question provides the opportunity for the man to advise you about how he is feeling and for you as the health professional to check your perceptions of how he is travelling. This also lets the man know that his level of distress is important to you. Feelings and levels of distress will vary over time depending on the challenges being faced. To keep track of how the participant is feeling from session to session, you will ask them to rate their current distress level at the beginning of each session.
- Ask the man to rate his average level of distress over the past week on a scale of 0 to 10.
- Anchor each end of the scale with a verbal descriptor (0 is no distress and 10 is the most distress he can imagine). You can also

refer him to a copy of the Distress Screen (including the Problem Checklist) for a visual reference.

- If he **reports a score of less than 4**, use the Problem Checklist as a guide and ask the man to nominate individual problems or concerns contributing to any distress. His answers will help guide your decision of which Flexible Component/s will be selected for the session.
- If he **reports a score of 4 or higher,** gently ask what is concerning him right now. Again, the Problem Checklist can be used as a guide. The nominated problems/challenges will help support the selection of the Flexible Component selected for the session. Reassure the man that it is sometimes upsetting to focus on and talk about cancer experiences but that, in the long run, it is usually helpful to discuss concerns. Using more in-depth screening tools (e.g., PHQ-9 and/or GAD-7), assess further for anxiety and depression and check for suicidal ideation or intention:
  - Assess if he is feeling **suicidal** (e.g., using the PHQ-9); if so, assess his level of risk and manage according to your service suicide response protocol. Manage suicidal ideation within your scope of practice and ethical responsibility.
- If on further screening the man reports **moderate to severe depression or anxiety** symptoms, this should be monitored for change during psychological care. In a stepped care approach, the focus or depth of care can then be adjusted to match the man's needs. The involvement of additional services such as a primary care physician or General Practitioner may be appropriate.

Additional Resources

- Prostate Cancer Distress Screen (Appendix 3)
- Prostate Cancer Survivorship Care Plan (Appendix 4)
- Patient Health Questionnaire (PHQ-9) (Appendix 5.1)
- Generalised Anxiety Disorder Assessment (GAD-7) (Appendix 5.2)

Distress screening training

- **University of Technology Sydney — Distress Screening for Prostate Cancer**: A free, self-paced online course that covers the nature and extent of psychological distress following prostate cancer, and distress screening. https://open.uts.edu.au/uts-open/study-area/health/distress-screening-for-prostate-cancer/
- **American Psychosocial Oncology Society (APOS) — Screening for Psychosocial Distress Program**: This program provides training to cancer care facilities on how to develop, implement, and maintain a comprehensive distress screening program. https://apos-society.org/professionals/distress-screening/psychosocial-distress-program-training/

Foundation Component Two: Agenda Setting

Agenda setting helps ensure clarity for both the health professional and the man on what the session will look like before it commences. Agreement is established about session goals guided by the man's priorities and the key care components identified by the health professional as important in addressing these priorities.

Agenda setting can be partly guided by the Prostate Cancer Distress Screen Problem Checklist on which men are encouraged to note down any problems or concerns that arise between sessions. Concerns raised by the man can then be reframed as priorities to address within the intervention session. What is most important however is to ask men to tell you about their main concerns and what they would like to change about their current situation.

A suggested format for agenda setting at the beginning of each session is as follows:

- **Encourage individual reflection**: Ask the man to discuss current concerns or problems related to his prostate cancer. These may already have been flagged using the Problem Checklist.
- **Confirm the nature of concern**: Reflect back to the man your understanding of what he most would like to change to ensure you are both on the same page.

- **Prioritise concerns**: If the man has several concerns discuss the order of importance of these concerns and establish with the man the priority for each to be addressed in the current session.
- **Reframe**: Guide the man in reframing their concerns into goals. Explain the importance of this step and how it will assist in making positive changes. Men can be asked 'What would you like to see instead?' in response to a concern or difficulty. For example, you might reframe 'I worry that I don't know what to do when I feel distressed' to 'Understanding my distress and how to manage these feelings'.
- **Evaluate goals**: Ensure goals are clear, realistic and achievable. For example, a goal of 'getting back to regular sex as soon as I can after surgery' could be changed to 'feeling comfortable in my intimate relationship'.
- **Problem solve**: Proceed to work towards goals using the problem-solving process (Flexible Component 5).

Homework

If this is the first session, or the first time you have introduced goal setting, suggest the man reads *Facing the Tiger* Chapter 2 — 'Why Me?' On Being Diagnosed With Prostate Cancer, and completes the goal setting activity on page 24 of the chapter prior to your next contact. To help him complete the activity you should provide him with a copy of **Tiger Activity Handout 2 — Goal Setting** (see Appendix 2.2).

Flexible Component 1

Psychoeducation – Coping with a Prostate Cancer Diagnosis

Introduction

Most people are unprepared for a cancer diagnosis. The difficult feelings and emotions that accompany a diagnosis can feel frightening and bewildering in and of themselves. Explaining why these emotions might occur and normalising this response (without minimising the importance of the problem) is the first key step.

Key Points

- The experience of a diagnosis of prostate cancer is a major life stress for men and their partners. That means its impact is going to be similar to other life stressors we may face, such as divorce, losing a job, or being in a serious accident.
- Cancer poses a threat to a person in two ways. First, cancer is potentially a threat to survival; and one of the first things many men think when they hear the word cancer is: 'How serious is this? Am

I going to die?' Cancer is also a threat to the 'self' — how we view ourselves. Men may wonder, 'How will this affect my life? Will I be the same person as I was before? Will I be able to do the things I usually do? How will my relationships change?'

- During this time, men may find they experience a range of difficult emotions and feelings, and they may not have felt this way before. This can range from feeling irritable or angry to feelings of loss of control and anxiety, and sometimes men even say, 'I felt like I was going crazy'.
- Partners often experience these emotions as well. However, everyone is different. A man's reaction to a prostate cancer diagnosis is his own. His partner and those close to him may not react in the same way.
- Thoughts, emotions, physical reactions, and behaviours or actions that are responses to the stressful event of a cancer diagnosis interact to influence how a person will cope with their individual cancer experience. This means that if a person becomes aware of their responses, they can apply strategies to manage these to ease distress and feel more in control (see Flexible Component 2: Stress management and wellbeing).
- It's important to know that cancer is not just one experience but a journey with different hurdles. There is the diagnosis itself, treatment decisions, recovering from treatment and managing treatment side-effects, and ongoing surveillance. Acknowledging the difficult aspects of prostate cancer and the loss and changes prostate cancer brings to the man's life is part of healing. It allows him to choose how to move forward.

Key Procedures

Coping styles and strategies

It is important for the man to understand his own personal coping style and consider adopting or developing new coping strategies that will help rather than hinder him. A recent systematic review reported that men tend to apply problem-solving coping when dealing with anxiety and utilise emotional self-reliance over formal help-seeking.[67] However, if problem-solving is not reducing or changing the problem, or if the problem can't be 'fixed', then a different approach is likely needed, and this might mean accepting or seeking formal help.

Most of us have our own typical approaches to problems or challenges. These are often learned in childhood, based on what our parents or peer-group told us or modelled by their own behaviour. For many men, this translates to expectations of being strong and stoic: don't cry when you are hurt; emotional suppression or keep your feelings to yourself; take risks; fight back; be self-reliant; and if it's broken, just fix it.

These approaches can make it harder for men to manage their health in the short and long term by bottling up difficult emotions and blocking support. In the face of a prostate cancer diagnosis, it is of course helpful for the man to adopt strategies that help him rather than hinder him. Thus he may need to change direction where coping is concerned. A helpful analogy here is to think about coping strategies as tools in a toolbox. In coping with cancer, they might have one tool they prefer, but if it doesn't seem to be working or getting the results they want, then another tool might make things a lot easier.
Coping approaches, or 'tools', are often put into two broad groups:

1. **Problem-solving coping**: This is an active approach that achieves outcomes and helps the man move forward in a practical and tangible way by applying strategies to solve the problem, for example, seeking different medical opinions or making a decision about which treatment to have.
2. **Emotion-focused coping**: This applies strategies to reduce painful or difficult emotions or feelings of distress, including talking to other people about how you feel, crying or expressing emotion, and using stress management and relaxation techniques. Emotion-focused coping strategies are a natural complement to problem-solving.

The ideal approach is to use flexible coping where the man is encouraged to change tack if his current approach is not working and is open to possibilities and change.

Discuss the things that are most stressful for the man currently about his cancer experience so far. It can be helpful to note these down on paper and draw them in a diagram to show how the man's thoughts, feelings, actions and physical responses are inter-relating. You may want to take him through part of the Activity on page 6 of *Facing the Tiger* using **Tiger Activity Handout 1 — Awareness of Responses to Stress and Coping Strategies**. (See Appendix 2.1)

- Draw a map on a piece of paper with four circles, one for thoughts, one for emotions, one for physical reactions and one for actions.
- Fill in examples in each box of what sort of thoughts, emotions, physical reactions and actions his stressors invoke.
- Ask about actions he took that were helpful? What did not work so well?
- Ask the man to think back to a different example in his life when he had a difficult time. Were his feelings then similar to now, or different? Does he have a typical way of coping with stress, and how well does that serve him?

Reinforce that the first step is awareness and understanding your own response, and accepting these are a natural reaction to a major life stress. The man might also find it helpful to discuss his response with a trusted friend, partner or adviser to help him start to process this experience and get clarity on his main concerns.

Homework

Suggest that the man:

- Read ***Facing the Tiger* Chapter 1**: Facing the Tiger, and ***Facing the Tiger* Chapter 2**: 'Why Me?' On Being Diagnosed With Prostate Cancer, prior to your next contact.
- If not already completed in the session, complete the *Facing the Tiger* chapter activity on page 6. You should provide a copy of **Tiger Activity Handout 1 — Awareness of Responses to Stress and Coping Strategies** for this activity (see Appendix 2.1).

If the man has a partner, ask if he is open to sharing the *Facing the Tiger* book with his partner. If the answer is yes, then suggest they read Chapter 3: 'Me too!' On Loving Someone With Prostate Cancer.

Assessment

Administer the *Prostate Cancer Distress Screen* at the start of the session (see Appendix 3) to inform and guide the session content. If the man scores at 4 or above on the Distress Scale, check for the presence of anxiety and/or depression, and suicidal ideation, and manage accordingly.

Key Resources

This component relates to *Facing the Tiger* Chapter 1: Facing the Tiger, and Chapter 2: 'Why Me?' On Being Diagnosed With Prostate Cancer.

Chapter 1 outlines the experience of cancer as a major life stress and introduces the premise of the book.

- **Activity**: (*Facing the Tiger* page 6) Awareness of responses to stress and coping strategies. Use **Tiger Activity Handout 1 — Awareness of Responses to Stress and Coping Strategies** in Appendix 2.1
- **Personal Stories:**

  David and Pam share the challenges they faced with prostate cancer and how they overcame these. They also share how the knowledge they gained from their own experience helped them to support their son when he was later diagnosed with prostate cancer at the age of 42 years.

  Gary talks about his experience from the perspective of a gay man and how he chose to face his cancer from a position of strength.

Chapter 2 explores reactions to a diagnosis of prostate cancer and different coping strategies, and introduces the concept of goal setting.

- **Activity**: (*Facing the Tiger* page 24) Goal Setting. Use **Tiger Activity Handout 2 — Goal Setting** in Appendix 2.2
- **Personal Stories:**

  Peter describes his experience with prostate cancer at a young age, the difficulties he faced after surgery, and the strategies he used to move forward.

Additional Resources

Consider following this component with *Flexible Component 2: Stress Management and Wellbeing*, to teach the man the importance of recognising and understanding his own stress response and using coping strategies effectively.

Flexible Component 2

Stress Management and Wellbeing

Introduction

A diagnosis of prostate cancer involves many different challenging situations. A man experiences stress when the demands of the challenges created by living with prostate cancer overwhelm his ability to cope with them. This component aims to teach the man to understand and recognise his own stress response and effectively use coping strategies to decrease the negative effects of stress and promote positive adjustment using relaxation and/or exercise. This component can be used to extend the information covered in *Flexible Component 1: Psychoeducation — Coping with a Prostate Cancer Diagnosis.*

Key Points

- To effectively manage stress, it is first of all important to know when you are experiencing stress. Stress awareness involves understanding the way your own body and mind reacts to significant challenges
- Coping refers to anything that we **do or think** to manage a challenging situation so that we don't become stressed or overwhelmed and/or to reduce our feelings of stress.

- We all have different ways of coping with challenging situations. These may be more or less helpful depending on whether our way of coping fits the demands of the situation.
- Some ways of coping that have been shown to be particularly helpful to people managing the effects of cancer include:
  - reducing the physical and emotional effects of stress using relaxation and/or exercise (covered in this component)
  - tackling the source of the stress by problem-solving (refer Flexible Component 5: Problem Solving)
  - challenging unhelpful thinking or changing how we react to thoughts (refer Flexible Component 6: Managing Difficult Thoughts)

Key Procedures

Review the Stress Response

Note that some men may not currently identify with any of the stress responses outlined. If this is the case, encourage them to relate to a past situation that they found particularly challenging. This will assist them to more personally identify with these responses.

Discuss common reactions to threatening or challenging situations, including:

- **Physical**: for example, increased heart rate, muscle tension, restlessness, nausea, chest tightness, sleeplessness.
- **Emotional**: for example, feeling irritable, anxious, angry, on edge, or frightened.
- **Behavioural**: for example, coping by withdrawing, keeping busy, sleeping/eating/drinking more than usual, trying to stay in control, snapping, talking more or less, information seeking.
- **Thoughts:** such as, *What if? What next?*

Suggest that it is normal to experience some degree of stress when faced with the challenges of prostate cancer. These challenges include the diagnosis, awaiting test results, dealing with treatment side effects, and coping with other people's reactions.

Ask the man about his particular reactions. If he finds this process difficult, ask him to close his eyes and visualise a stressful situation such as locking his keys in the car or waiting in a traffic jam when late for an appointment.

Work with him to generate a list of his physical, emotional, thinking and behavioural reactions to such a situation. You may again want to take him through the Activity on page 6 of *Facing the Tiger* using **Tiger Activity Handout 1 — Awareness of Responses to Stress and Coping Strategies** (See Appendix 2.1)

- Draw a map on a piece of paper with four circles, one for thoughts, one for emotions, one for physical reactions and one for actions.
- Fill in examples in each box of what sort of thoughts, emotions, physical reactions and actions his stressors invoke.
- Ask about actions he took that were helpful? What did not work so well?
- Ask the man to think back to a different example in his life when he had a difficult time. Were his feelings then similar to now, or different? Does he have a typical way of coping with stress, and how well does that serve him?

Discuss how these stress responses are linked to each other. For example, thinking scary/angry thoughts can lead to increased bodily tension and feelings of anxiety or anger. Where possible, use the man's personal experiences to demonstrate the relationship between thoughts, feelings, physical reactions and coping. Use positive as well as negative examples, for example, feeling anxious can lead to increased energy which leads to increased motivation to seek answers or speak to others. Regular exercise that leads to a decrease in scary thoughts helps you feel less anxious.

Outline the Benefits of Relaxation Strategies

Relaxation is not simply recreation, rest, or leisure time. It is also not daydreaming or letting your mind wander. Learning to relax involves becoming aware of reactions to stress and knowing when you need to take time out to reduce tension. Deep relaxation is a learned skill and involves the knowledge and skill to induce the *relaxation response* by consciously focusing on relaxing your mind and body. The *relaxation response* counteracts the effects of stress in the body and has been proven to lower heart rate and blood pressure and improve general wellbeing. It takes practice to learn to induce the *relaxation response*, and the techniques are best practised daily.

Include in your discussion:

- The importance of relaxation as a strategy in the reduction of physical and mental tension and thereby reducing other symptoms of stress as well (i.e., using the *relaxation response* to counteract the stress response).
- Suggest that relaxation exercises offer the added benefit of helping the man to:
  - recognise when he is tense; and
  - reduce stress in situations such as doctor's waiting rooms, workplace or bed, when other strategies may prove impossible to implement.

When a person feels overwhelmed, it can be difficult to break the cycle of tension or anxiety they feel. Relaxation exercises enable a person to stop, slow things down, and focus on reducing their feelings of stress.

Review Relaxation Practices

- Brainstorm strategies the man may have used in the past to relax, e.g., walking, exercise, listening to music, meditation, or spending time in the garden.
- Introduce the brief relaxation exercise outlined on pages 93–94 of *Facing the Tiger* and provide the man with a copy of the **Tiger Relaxation Handout** (see Appendix 2.3). Explain that controlling and slowing your breath is a very simple way to calm your body, that breathing techniques are easy to do anywhere and anytime, and because they are not obvious to those around you, they can be done in almost any situation of stress.
- Ask the man to sit comfortably and focus for a few minutes on being aware of his breathing, then talk him through the following:
  - Notice how your breath moves in and out of your nose and chest and how your chest muscles contract and relax as you breathe.
  - Listen to the sound of your breath as you breathe in and out.
  - Be aware of your posture and how your shoulders sit as you breathe. If your shoulders are tight and hunched, drop them down on your out-breath.
  - Next, count slowly to four in every in and out-breath you take. Focus your mind on the count, and breathe in a slow and relaxed

  and comfortable way in time to the count. Do this for several minutes as your body gets used to slow and controlled breathing.
  - Now stop and notice how you feel.
- This is a quick and easy de-stress strategy that can be easily applied to good effect when stuck in traffic, waiting in a doctor's office for a check-up, or at night just before going to sleep to relax yourself down. This exercise can be extended by adding in at the end:
  - For a few breaths only, hold your breath for a count of two.
  - You can also add visualisation or imagery by asking the man to focus his mind on a safe and relaxing scenario or image once his breathing has slowed down.
  - This might mean building a picture in his mind of a relaxing place and activity, such as swimming in the sea or walking in a forest, and imagining the colours and sounds and physical sensations he would experience if he were there.
- Suggest that this is a quick, easy and portable strategy for use in any situation that triggers tension.
- Discuss the importance of regular relaxation practice (e.g., 15 mins daily) in contributing to an overall reduction in levels of arousal as well as helping them in stressful situations. Suggest that, like any new skill, it takes time and practice, and they will need to dedicate time individually to mastering this strategy.
- Pre-empt that often, when faced with the challenges of cancer diagnosis and treatment, people find it difficult to take the time to relax. Discuss the benefit of scheduling regular times to learn to induce the *relaxation response* — suggest scheduling times in the diary or calendar as a reminder.
- If the man appears open to trying another approach to relaxation you might like to take them through the mindfulness focussing activity on pages 96–97 of *Facing the Tiger* and provide him with a copy of the **Tiger Activity Handout 3 — Mindfulness Focussing** (see Appendix 2.4).

Exercise and stress management

For many men, exercise is their preferred way to reduce physical and mental stress. They feel comfortable with the approach, and exercise is generally associated with better psychological wellbeing. The benefits of exercise for cancer care are widely acknowledged.[68,69] For men with prostate cancer, it is recommended they seek advice from an Accredited Exercise Physiologist, or equivalent, to be assessed and prescribed a targeted exercise program for even greater effectiveness.[70] The Godin-Shephard Leisure-Time Physical Activity Questionnaire[71] is a 3-item tool that can be used to assess physical activity levels of men with prostate cancer.

Include in your discussion:

- Exercise has been proven, through extensive research, to significantly improve physical and mental health for men with prostate cancer, and ecological data suggests it may also improve prostate cancer survival.
- Appropriate exercise has been proven to be very safe for men with prostate cancer, including those with advanced disease.[72]
- Men are now being encouraged to exercise in the weeks before surgery to build their resilience and following surgery to advance recovery.
- Exercising while on testosterone suppression or hormone-blocking treatment helps to reduce side effects such as fat gain and muscle and bone loss.
- During and after treatment, exercise can improve urinary control and sexual function, reduce fatigue and tiredness, improve sleep, help with balance and reduce the risk of falls, and is associated with better thinking.
- Before starting a new exercise program, it is important to have a health check with your doctor and get advice from an Accredited Exercise Physiologist.
- An Accredited Exercise Physiologist can tailor a program to your needs and goals that include both strengthening (resistance) and aerobic (cardio) exercise.
- As a general rule, you need to exercise for twenty to sixty minutes at least three times a week to get a meaningful benefit. The intensity should be moderate to vigorous.

You may like to take the man through the Activity on page 100 of *Facing the Tiger* if prioritising exercise is a session goal. Provide him with a copy of **Tiger Activity Handout 4 — Goal Setting to De-stress** (see Appendix 2.5) and help him work through the activity as follows:

- Ask the man how he feels most of the time and if he feels there is room for improvement in the way he looks after himself.

- Use the following checklist as a start and prioritise which of these things he would most like to work on.
    - Exercising more
    - Feeling calmer
    - Reducing my weight
    - Feeling stronger physically
    - Any other ways?
- Identify his goals, the short and medium-term milestones he wants to reach, and when he expects to get there.
- Have him list the steps he will need to take to move towards these milestones:
    - who and what he needs to help him achieve these
    - what barriers he might need to address
- Ask him to pick a date to get started
- Reassure him that setbacks are normal and to watch for unhelpful 'all or nothing' thinking. Most things that are worthwhile are effort, but if he never starts, he most certainly will not get there

Homework

Suggest the man:

- Read ***Facing the Tiger* Chapter 8**: De-Stressing: How to Look After Yourself and Keep Well, prior to your next contact
- Try the mindfulness activity on page 96 of *Facing the Tiger*.
- If not completed in the session, complete the *Facing the Tiger* activity Prioritising Exercise for De-stressing on page 100. You should provide a copy of **Tiger Activity Handout 4 — Goal Setting to De-stress** for this activity (see Appendix 2.5).

Assessment

Administer the *Prostate Cancer Distress Screen* at the start of the session (see Appendix 3) to inform and guide the session content. If the man scores at 4 or above on the Distress Scale, check for the presence of anxiety and/or depression, and suicidal ideation, and manage accordingly.

Key Resources

This component relates to *Facing the Tiger* Chapter 8: De-Stressing: How to Look After Yourself and Keep Well.

Chapter 8 outlines how to reduce physical and mental tension, provides strategies for relaxation and discusses the role of exercise in reducing stress and supporting wellbeing.

- **Activity:** (*Facing the Tiger* page 96) Mindfulness Focussing. Use **Tiger Activity Handout 3 — Mindfulness Focussing** in Appendix 2.4.
- **Activity:** (*Facing the Tiger* page 100) Goal Setting to De-stress. Use **Tiger Activity Handout 4 — Goal Setting to De-stress** in Appendix 2.5.
- **Personal Stories:**

  Charles talks about how he came to take up an exercise program to help with prostate cancer treatment side effects that has turned into a normal way of life for him and his partner.

  Jan and Gordon talk about how they use mindfulness and breathing techniques to manage stress.

  Roger talks about how he got into dragon boating and how this has enhanced his fitness and his social life.

  Patrick explains how he maintains his physical and psychological health through exercise, meditation and the pursuit of knowledge.

Additional Resources

The Godin-Shephard Leisure-Time Physical Activity Questionnaire: https://www.ons.org/sites/default/files/Godin%20Leisure-Time%20Exercise%20Questionnaire_070815.pdf

For other approaches to stress management, consider:

- **Flexible Component 5: Problem Solving** to tackle the source of the stress by problem-solving
- **Flexible Component 6: Managing Difficult Thoughts** for challenging unhelpful thinking.

Flexible Component 3

Treatment Decision Making

Introduction

Men are often surprised to find that there is a choice to be made about the type of treatment they receive for prostate cancer and that the doctors want to involve them in making the decision. These include the complexity of medical terms and jargon that are difficult for many people to understand, the stress and anxiety associated with a prostate cancer diagnosis, the challenge of interpreting treatment and cancer-related risks, and lay understandings about cancer and cancer treatment.

Applying a systematic approach can help men navigate decision making with the goal of making a decision where they understand the potential risks and benefits and how these connect to their own personal preferences and values, and are confident about their choice.

Key Points

- The idea that one way to treat a cancer is to keep a close watch rather than actively treat the disease goes against the messages we usually hear about cancer.
- Many men expect doctors to advise one particular action to take, so finding out that there is no single right way can be confusing.

- The information about prostate cancer treatments often includes difficult medical terms and statistics and can be hard to understand.
- Each of the treatment options has potentially serious negative outcomes for the man.
- Most men feel anxious just about having cancer, and this can make it harder to think decisions through.

Key Procedures

Decision Making

There are steps men can use to help themselves in their decision making. For men who have already made a decision, these steps help ensure that they have all the information they need to be prepared for treatment. These steps can also be applied to decisions in the future and so can be helpful in that way.

The Ottawa Personal Decision Guide[73] proposes four decision steps for making decisions about health and can be used to work through difficult decisions systematically. The steps include:

1. ***Being clear*** about the decision
2. Being as ***involved*** in the decision as you wish and get helpful support
3. Considering the ***pros and cons*** and weighing the options
4. ***Planning*** the next steps.

Being Clear about the Decision

If you judge that high levels of distress (e.g., due to high cancer threat appraisal or other stressors) are interfering with the man's ability to make a decision, it is important to assess the reason for his distress. This might include high levels of arousal due to appraisal of the cancer as highly threatening, or preoccupation with other stressors he perceives as equally or more important. It is important to address the high levels of distress using relevant stress management strategies (e.g., thought challenging, relaxation, problem-solving) in order to help the man find the cognitive space to think through his decision.

Once the man has clarified the decision he faces and how far along he is with his decision, focussed decision support can be provided. This may include:

- **Discussing the treatment options** his doctor has suggested and his understanding of the reasons why he has these options. Ask the man what he has been thinking about in making his decision. Check for inaccurate perceptions or beliefs about cancer that may be influencing his choice and gently challenge these where necessary and/or clarify points of uncertainty or misunderstanding.

- **Checking and confirming** that the man has relevant patient education materials at hand and direct the man to the materials that most closely meet his needs, depending upon his level of literacy and his preferences for information. If the man has not yet reviewed these educational resources suggest that he might find it useful to read or view them before his next doctor's appointment. Reassure the man that usually with prostate cancer there is no need to hurry with the decision about treatment. This means he can take time to reach a decision that he is confident with. Suggest the man confirm this with his doctor.

Decision Support

Discuss with the man how he would prefer to decide about treatment. Review with him that an important contributor to decision satisfaction is having the support that he prefers in making this decision. Suggest that many men prefer to share the decision equally with their doctor and that some men will want decision support from their partner. Some men find peer support groups helpful. Still others may prefer to think the decision through on their own after listening to their doctors' advice.

Whilst some men may not want to discuss their decision with their partner, for others, this will be important. Partners have the potential to play an important supporting role. For example, they can help with seeking and interpreting information and reassuring the man that despite his cancer and the possible treatment side effects, he is still loved and valued. The effects of treatment on sexual function will have a significant impact on the partner and the man, so encouraging partner participation in the man's care from the time of decision-making is important.

Consider the pros and cons of the different options

If a man has already read through the patient education material, considered his treatment options and discussed these with his doctor and support persons as desired, he may be ready to proceed to considering the pros and cons. If he is not yet clear about his options, it will be more helpful for him to first read the patient education materials and then talk with his doctor about his options before proceeding. A question list may help him to focus on his areas of uncertainty. Scheduling time to talk to relevant family members about the decision may also be helpful.

The next step will be to consider the pros and cons of each of the treatment options available to him, thinking about his own personal preferences and values — what is important to him personally.

Using the Decision Guide

Offer to work through the Decision Guide with the man as follows:

- For each treatment option he is considering, ask him to generate positives and negatives from his individual point of view.
- Encourage the man to rate the relative importance of each of his listed positives and negatives.
- He may find it useful to use a star system such as 1 star = low importance, 5 stars = high importance.
- Support the man to look at the relative balance of the positives and negatives for each option and see if he can observe where he is leaning towards in his decision
- Suggest that he discuss this list with his doctor at his next visit.

Homework

Suggest the man:

- Read ***Facing the Tiger* Chapter 5**: How to Make Decisions You Can Live With, prior to your next contact.
- Complete the *Facing the Tiger* activity on page 58 on treatment decision making. You should provide a copy of **Tiger Activity Handout 5 — Treatment Decision Making** for this activity (see Appendix 2.6).

Assessment

Administer the *Prostate Cancer Distress Screen* at the start of the session (see Appendix 3) to inform and guide the session content. If the man scores at 4 or above on the Distress Scale, check for the presence of anxiety and/or depression, and suicidal ideation, and manage accordingly.

Key Resources

This component relates to *Facing the Tiger* Chapter 5: How to Make decisions you can Live With.

Chapter 5 outlines how to make decisions when under stress.

- **Activity:** (Facing the Tiger page 58) Treatment Decision Making. Use **Tiger Activity Handout — Treatment Decision Making** in Appendix 2.6.
- **Personal Stories:**

  Geoff and Allan share how they each approached making their decisions about treatment and how they feel about that decision now.

Additional Resources

- **Ottawa Personal Decision Guide:**

  https://decisionaid.ohri.ca/docs/das/OPDG.pdf

Distress related to decision making should be managed using relevant stress management strategies:

- **Flexible Component 2: Stress Management and Wellbeing** to help with relaxation strategies.
- **Flexible Component 5: Problem Solving** to manage distress by problem-solving.
- **Flexible Component 6: Managing Difficult Thoughts** for challenging unhelpful thinking.

Flexible Component 4

Managing Relationships Under Stress

Introduction

Strong social support is an important coping resource and buffers an individual from the negative effects of a stressful event. From this, it follows that good family and/or partner support is especially important for an individual's wellbeing when they are facing a cancer diagnosis. A diagnosis of cancer is a major life stress not only for the man but also for his partner, and relationships can be strained by this experience, sometimes in a way couples and families have not felt before. If a man does not have a partner, then support from other close family or friends will be important. In this situation, finding ways to show and share support, understand differences and communicate effectively about what is happening is crucial. Above all, it remains important for the health professional to understand and work within the relationship context of the man and what is appropriate and acceptable for him and those close to him.

Key Points

This component contains information and strategies to increase support and communication after prostate cancer for couples and close family or friends. The three parts have been designed to stand alone or be grouped into a more comprehensive session. To increase engagement, it starts with information and strategies likely to be viewed as most relevant to participants. It is followed by other evidence-based strategies demonstrated to increase relationship satisfaction. These may not be relevant for those who do not perceive that they need relationship enhancement.

- **Part 1: Showing Support**: This is designed to increase the mutual support that partners offer each other over the course of diagnosis, treatment and post-treatment. The anticipated outcome of this part is the facilitation of adjustment through increased support and decreased helplessness. Men are prompted to think and talk about emotional and practical ways of supporting their partner.
- **Part 2: Understanding Differences**: This helps men to understand and more effectively manage any misunderstandings that might arise when dealing with a stressful life event such as a prostate cancer diagnosis. Men are asked to identify patterns of managing conflict and set ground rules for managing disagreements.
- **Part 3: Talking to Each Other:** This assists men to communicate more effectively about cancer-related challenges, maximising support and minimising the potential for withdrawal and/or conflict. During the session men can gain an understanding of their current communication patterns. The health professional also reviews key elements of good communication and provides training in basic communication skills.

Key Procedures

Part 1: Showing Support

This part assists men to identify ways to support the people affected by their diagnosis, practically and emotionally, through the challenges of prostate cancer. It focuses on providing a rationale for communicating support needs, exploring ways of showing support that have (and have not) been effective to date, and consideration by men of how they would most like to be supported by the people in their lives.

Describe the rationale for identifying ways to show support by including the following points in your discussion.

- The availability of good support is important for how men and their loved one's cope with the challenges of prostate cancer.

- People sometimes cope with the problems of diagnosis and treatment by keeping busy and getting on with things — giving little consideration to how they are feeling or the sort of support they would like.
- Many people don't like to ask for support (even if they know what they want) because they want to protect those around them from extra burdens.
- Not knowing how to support each other can *increase* feelings of helplessness, distress, and loneliness.
- Ask the man to identify how they have been showing support to their partner over the past few weeks and in what ways this has been helpful or not so helpful.

Part 2: Understanding Differences

The focus of this part is to assist men to understand and manage differences. It provides information about different ways of coping with prostate cancer and encourages men to consider their own individual ways of coping. The purpose is to support the acceptance of differences and find ways to manage these.

You should first **provide a rationale** for exploring how to deal with these differences by including the following points in your discussion.

- One reason that people may find it difficult to know how to support each other is the fact that they are different. Every person is different in their personality and ways of coping. These differences often become more obvious in times of high stress, such as coping with a cancer diagnosis.
- Some people cope by sharing their fears and sadness openly with others. Talking things through can help them to feel less alone and more in control.
- Other people prefer to cope by thinking about cancer as little as possible. They may prefer to keep busy to distract themselves from negative thoughts or feelings.
- Sometimes a person may switch between wanting to talk about things at one time and then wanting to avoid difficult thoughts and feelings at another time.
- Often people can find it difficult to feel close to one another if one person wants to talk and the other does not. This can lead to misunderstandings and avoidance.

Part 3: Talking to each other

The focus of this part is to enhance communication. It provides guidance in key communication skills and encourages men to consider how they can routinely use these skills to manage the stress of the cancer diagnosis. The primary goal is to assist men in finding ways to speak and listen to those around them more effectively.

Discuss the rationale for maintaining or enhancing good communication by including the following points in your discussion.

- Most people have ways of communicating that generally work well for them. Maintaining or enhancing good communication can help men to navigate prostate cancer.
- Sometimes men find they are talking less after prostate cancer is diagnosed. Less communication during times of stress may be a familiar pattern to some men. For others it is a new or unusual experience.
- Factors that can make it more difficult to come together to talk include:
    - Being too busy with the increased demands on your time, e.g., getting things done at work or around the house, attending doctor's appointments, etc.
    - Not knowing what you think or feel or not knowing how to put it into words
    - A belief that there is no point talking or involving your partner as they won't really understand
    - A belief that involving your partner may make things worse
    - Not wanting to get upset yourself by talking about difficult issues
    - Not wanting to upset the other person by bringing things up
- Not talking to those around you or withdrawing can lead to increased stress as the others can feel increasingly 'shut out' and/or may misinterpret or misjudge your actions. This can lead to increased conflict and/or significant others just 'giving up'.
- Withdrawing also makes it very difficult for your support people to know how to provide you with support. This not only makes it more difficult for you to get the support you want but leads to increased feelings of helplessness for others.

- We often think we know our partners so well that we also know what they are thinking — mind reading. Alternatively, expecting another person to mind-read, that is, to know our needs or understand our feelings without our having to tell them.

Discuss whether the man recognises any of these unhelpful communication patterns.

Review strategies to enhance or improve communication including the following points in your discussion.

- It is important to recognise and accept each other's differences and coping styles and accept them. Suggest that it is unlikely to help if one partner blows up because the other partner will not always talk about his feelings. Consider that they might have a greater need to spend time alone or to think through solutions.
- If one partner needs to explore his or her feelings and the other partner is not a talker, then it may help to instead confide in a close friend or to join a support group. Another way to explore your feelings is to write about them.
- It might be useful to set aside times when you both agree to talk about the cancer and how you are each managing, and then at other times focus on your broader life and future plans and shared interests.

If the man is ready to make time to talk to his partner, talk him through the following strategies.

- Make a dedicated time to come together to talk about how you are both managing with the challenges you currently face or any present concerns.
- When choosing a time, consider:
    - This time is just for the two of you, so minimise distractions or interruptions. For example, make sure the television is turned off and don't answer the phone or look at your mobile messages.
    - Choose a time when you are both likely to be relaxed and able to concentrate on each other. Avoid trying to talk together if either of you is very tired. You may end up saying things you do not mean.

- Take the man through the steps of the *Facing the Tiger* activity on page 43 and help him work through the activity as follows:
  - Set aside about 20 minutes once or twice a week to talk with each other about how you each are feeling and coping.
  - No problem solving, just listening and making sure you have checked you understand and 'get it'.
  - Don't judge or criticise and don't interrupt.
  - Think of three to five things your partner could do to support you. Make a commitment to each other to try these out and see how it goes. Be clear about which support action matters the most to each of you.
  - Take time to do a pleasurable activity with each other that has nothing to do with cancer.

Homework

Suggest that the man:

- Read ***Facing the Tiger* Chapter 4**: We're in This Together, prior to your next contact.
- Complete the *Facing the Tiger* activity on page 43, which focuses on setting aside time to talk.

Assessment

Administer the *Prostate Cancer Distress Screen* at the start of the session (see Appendix 3) to inform and guide the session content. If the man scores at 4 or above on the Distress Scale, check for the presence of anxiety and/or depression, and suicidal ideation, and manage accordingly.

Key Resources

This component relates to *Facing the Tiger* Chapter 4: We're in This Together.

Chapter 4 outlines how prostate cancer affects partners and families and how everyone copes differently. It also provides practical strategies for communicating with your partner, especially if their coping strategies differ from your own.

- **Personal Stories**:

  Jan and Gordon talk about how weekly meetings helped them keep in touch with what was going on for each other.

  Jim and Laura found that being patient and accepting each other as they are was crucial.

  Casey talks about how he and his partner worked together as a team and have been able to maintain their intimacy as well as respect for each other's space.

Flexible Component 5

Problem Solving

Introduction

A problem-solving approach to intervening with men is based on the premise that cancer is a major negative life event that can result in a number of stressful situations. The consequences of being diagnosed with advanced prostate cancer can leave the men feeling regret about treatment decisions, uncertainty/fear about the future, low self-esteem with regards to their masculinity and concerns about ongoing treatment effects, all of which can lead to lasting distress. It is hypothesised that distress is more likely to occur if the demands of a situation/s overwhelm the man's coping efforts.

It is important to note that men facing prostate cancer treatment will experience differing levels of distress depending on their *unique* cancer-related problems and their ability to cope with these problems. However, it is assumed that there are some problems (or potential problems) that will be shared by most men facing prostate cancer.

Key Points

The focus of this component is to teach men a **5-step problem-solving process** that they can use to eliminate or modify sources of stress in their lives. It can prove especially helpful in assisting men in managing practical challenges associated with prostate cancer treatments.

Introduce the rationale for problem-solving by including the following points in your discussion.

- Prostate cancer and its treatment can raise a number of challenges that may add to already existing problems.
- When we are distressed, problems seem overwhelming and insurmountable. This can lead to increased distress and make the problems worse.
- Structured problem solving helps us to focus on what we can do about issues rather than just worrying about them.
- Problem solving is a way of working logically through obstacles — breaking them down into more manageable chunks and helping men feel more in control.
- You can use 5 steps that can be applied either to practical problems such as how to manage household demands while having daily radiotherapy or to interpersonal problems such as how to resolve a conflict.
- Problem solving can improve a man's ability to manage the challenges of prostate cancer, decrease the distress associated with these and other problems, improve quality of life, and increase a sense of control over health and life generally.

Key Procedures

The **5 sequential steps of problem-solving** include:

1. **Define the problem**. Be clear about what the problem is and find accurate information from reputable sources about the issue so that you understand why it has arisen and what it means.
2. **Brainstorm**. Generate different options or possibilities for dealing with the problem. The more alternative solutions you generate, the better. The point is to come up with as many different ideas as possible.
3. **Evaluate solutions**. Evaluate the pros and cons of each possible solution. This should include what help you might need and from whom, how confident you feel about each approach working for you.
4. **Select the 'best' option and make a plan**. Pick the option that looks best and has the best chance of successfully solving or managing the

problem. The plan needs to be clear about the steps you will need to take — the 'who', 'what', 'when', 'where', and 'how' of the plan. Include a timeline for each step.

5. **Take action and evaluate the outcome**. Be clear about what success would mean for this problem and how you will evaluate for yourself how you have gone. Be prepared to re-evaluate your plan and adjust or change it if it isn't working for you. Having a flexible approach is crucial.

Review Problem Solving Strategies

Use the results of the Problem Checklist (see Appendix 3) from the distress screening at the start of the session, or an envisaged problem (practical or personal), to work through an example together. If the man finds it difficult to identify a problem themselves, suggest reflecting on any situation that has led them to feel strong negative feelings, for example, feeling overwhelmed, frightened, angry, depressed.

Homework

Suggest that the man:

- Read **Facing the Tiger Chapter 9**: Solving Problems After Treatment, prior to your next contact
- Read the examples of applying a problem-solving approach on page 113 of *Facing the Tiger* (fatigue and getting back to work) and 116 of *Facing the Tiger* (solving urinary problems) and think about how they might relate to the man's own situation.
- Complete the *Facing the Tiger* problem-solving activity on page 119. You should provide a copy of **Tiger Activity Handout 6 — Problem Solving** for this activity (See Appendix 2.7).

Assessment

Administer the *Prostate Cancer Distress Screen* at the start of the session (see Appendix 3) to inform and guide the session content. If the man scores at 4 or above on the Distress Scale, check for the presence of anxiety and/or depression, and suicidal ideation, and manage accordingly.

Key Resources

This component relates to *Facing the Tiger* Chapter 9: Solving Problems After Treatment.

Chapter 9 outlines the problem-solving steps and provides practical examples of problem-solving applied to managing fatigue to return to work and solving urinary problems.

- **Activity**: (*Facing the Tiger* page 119) Problem Solving. Use **Tiger Activity Handout 6 — Problem Solving** in Appendix 2.7.
- **Personal Stories:**

  Norman shares how he approached problems he faced after prostate cancer treatment. This included getting outside support with the help of his son Tristan when things got very tough.

  Gerry talks about how he was a bit too chilled out after treatment.

  Graham shares how a very tough time turned around once he got the right advice.

Flexible Component 6

Managing Difficult Thoughts

Introduction

In earlier components, we outlined a stress and cancer model and the importance of being aware of the interaction between thoughts, emotions, physical reactions and actions. In this component the focus is on the central role of our thoughts and how we respond to them; how they influence our experience not only of stressful events, but of life more broadly. An important aspect of this session is to encourage the man to see thoughts as 'just thoughts' rather than 'facts'. A skill to learn here is for men to become aware of their thought patterns and look at them with curiosity and interest rather than react and respond to them as if they were automatically true.

Key Points

Thought Challenging

Once a person becomes aware of their thoughts, one way to manage the distress response is to challenge the thoughts and look for alternative approaches or ways to think about the situation. Suppressing or avoiding difficult thoughts tends to not work in the long run and is exhausting.

Introduce the concept of thought challenging by including the following points in your discussion.

- The way we think about situations strongly influences how we feel and respond.
- Some thoughts help a person feel and cope better, while other thoughts may cause them to be more distressed and prevent them from coping effectively.
- The thoughts we have in a stressful situation are often 'automatic' in that we may not even be aware we are thinking them.
- When we are under stress, our automatic thoughts are often unbalanced. They may be overly negative (e.g., 'the side effects will be unbearable', 'my wife will not cope'), may overestimate your problems (e.g., 'everything will go wrong', 'my health is shot to pieces'), or may not be based on a realistic assessment of the evidence (e.g., 'a delay in test results means bad news', 'I have let everyone down').
- Overly negative, self-blaming thinking results in the person feeling even more upset and finding it even harder to cope with an already difficult situation.

Key Procedures

Thinking Patterns

Introduce the concept of thinking patterns by including the following points in your discussion.

- Thinking patterns develop from a young age and are based on the messages we received as we grew up. For example, if the main message was that the world was not a safe place, the way we think and feel may be hyper-vigilant for danger or punishment. Conversely, if we were told that things would generally work out okay, we might be less likely to jump to the worst conclusions.
- Neither way is better or worse but predicting or assuming the worst a lot of the time contributes to distress.
- Some common but unhelpful thinking patterns people use include:
    - **Catastrophising**: thinking of the worst possible outcome that could happen.

- **Black and White Thinking** (also called 'all or nothing thinking' or 'my way or the highway'): thinking that things have to go a certain way or it will be a complete disaster.
- **Self-blame**: thinking that it is all your fault.
- **Overgeneralising**: taking one event and turning it into a sweeping generalisation about how things will always be.
- **The Negative Mental Filter**: seeing only the negative aspects of a situation and ignoring all of the positives.
- **Jumping to Conclusions**: assuming something is negative when there is actually not much evidence to support it.

Review Thought Challenging Strategies

Discuss that the first step in challenging unhelpful thoughts is to recognise what you are thinking or saying to yourself. Suggest that one way of knowing you are thinking in a negative way is when you are distressed, for example, feeling scared, anxious, depressed, or angry.

- Ask the man to think about a recent situation where he felt upset or stressed and to identify his thoughts at the time.
- Assist the man to assess the validity of these thoughts in a more balanced way:
    - What are the **facts** in this situation? Is the way I am thinking consistent with the facts?
    - What is the **evidence** that this thought or view is 100% true and correct?
    - Is this a **realistic** thought? Is this really likely to happen? How likely is it to happen?
    - Is thinking in this way **helping or hindering** me from coping and feeling better or achieving a positive outcome?
    - What is the **effect** of thinking this way? What are the consequences?

Review strategies for replacing unrealistic/unhelpful thoughts with alternative, more helpful ways to think about the problem/situation:

- What are some **alternative** ways of thinking about this or possible alternative explanations for what happened?
- What is a more **realistic** way to think about it?

- What is a more **helpful** way to think about it?
- What would I **tell a mate** if he were in a similar situation?

Suggest that in order for him to challenge his thoughts effectively, his new thought must be believable.

Discuss that it is not helpful to deny that cancer is serious or frightening, and trying to think overly positive thoughts and putting on a brave face all the time can be an emotional drain. The man needs to encourage or 'coach' himself through difficulties rather than be critical and undermining. In this sense, he needs to learn to be a good mate or friend to himself.

Encourage Ongoing Use of Thought Challenging

Suggest the man use Thought Challenging strategies to help him to cope with strong negative feelings over the next several weeks. Suggest that, like any new skill, it takes time to feel comfortable and confident using it. Reassure him that the more he practices, the more he will automatically start to use this skill.

Homework

Suggest that the man:

- Read ***Facing the Tiger* Chapter** 7. I think therefore I am, prior to your next contact
- Complete the *Facing the Tiger* activity on page 82 on automatic thinking. You should provide a copy of **Tiger Activity Handout 7— Automatic Thinking** for this activity (see Appendix 2.8).
- Complete the *Facing the Tiger* activity on page 86 on identifying patterns of thinking. You should provide a copy of **Tiger Activity Handout 8 — Identifying Patterns of Thinking** for this activity (see Appendix 2.9).

Assessment

Administer the *Prostate Cancer Distress Screen* at the start of the session (see Appendix 3) to inform and guide the session content. If the man scores at 4 or above on the Distress Scale, check for the presence of anxiety and/or depression, and suicidal ideation, and manage accordingly.

Key Resources

This component relates to *Facing the Tiger* Chapter 7: I think therefore I am.

Chapter 7 outlines how thought processes work and some common thinking patterns that can emerge under stress.

- **Activity**: (*Facing the Tiger* page 82) Automatic Thinking. Use **Tiger Activity Handout 7 — Automatic Thinking** in Appendix 2.8.
- **Activity**: (*Facing the Tiger* page 86) Identifying Patterns of Thinking. Use **Tiger Activity Handout 8 — Identifying Patterns of Thinking** in Appendix 2.9.
- **Personal Stories**:

  David shares his prostate cancer experience and how he has learnt to manage worrying thoughts and keep stress under control.

Flexible Component 7

Pivoting to Valued Directions

Introduction

The experience of prostate cancer and the stresses associated with this, including for some men permanent changes in physical functioning, can exacerbate long-standing but unhelpful ways of being. For example, if a person has had a tendency towards excessive self-blame or negative self-judgement, avoidant coping approaches, or rumination and worry, then experiencing cancer may focus a spotlight on this way of being. Such a tendency to cope and to persevere in these ways has been conceptualised as **psychological rigidity**. Psychological rigidity represents patterns of responses that aim to avoid pain but paradoxically serve to sustain it.[45]

Through understanding and being aware of their response to prostate cancer, men may also find that an awareness of their patterns of psychological rigidity emerges, and from this, a desire for change may arise. Developing a non-judgemental awareness of well-practised habits of responses to life events and relationships is a good starting point to support this change. From this approach, a person can potentially move towards an acceptance of these as part of their life journey (though not necessarily as the director of the future) and then move to pay attention to the present moment and experience. In the present moment a person may choose to review their life values, what is most important to them now, and then set behavioural goals to pivot towards these values and valued ways of living. For each man this is a choice that they can make within the bounds of the resources they have within themselves and that they have available externally to call on. Once these values are clear, the man can identify behaviours they can work towards. The key is to flexibly adapt their approach to achieving what they most desire and ideally have harmony between their valued directions and their life choices and patterns. This is termed **psychological flexibility**. If such an approach fits with the type of support and change the man is seeking, there are many self-help materials that discuss this in more detail.[45,74]

Key Points

Introduce the concept of psychological flexibility by including the following points in your discussion.

- The first step is self-awareness without judgement of feelings and thoughts the man may be experiencing that are uncomfortable or distressing. Most people will tend to avoid difficult feelings and thoughts and so allowing space for these to be noticed in a self-compassionate stance is crucial.
- Once these difficult feelings and thoughts are recognised, explore with the man the origin of these, how he might have learnt this way of responding, and what the consequences have been for him.
- To help the man look at these feelings and thoughts without judgement, you might ask him to consider if he had a close friend or someone he cared about in this situation, what would he see? What advice would he give to himself if he was his own best and trusted friend?
- The next step is working out how he wants to be and identifying the key areas of his life hat he would like to change, and conversely, what is holding him back.
- Finally, planning behavioural change and scheduling actions to work on with complete commitment is the step that moves to change. The aim is for the man to experiment in widening out the range and view of what is possible in his life.
- Above all, though, change is a personal choice, and for the health professional there must also be no judgement. Change is hard. Most people are doing the best they can to live a good and productive life. Supporting personal agency in the choices the man

makes about his future wellbeing means exactly that. He gets to choose in awareness of his present being and in accordance with his personal values and preferences.

Homework

Suggest that the man:

- Read ***Facing the Tiger* Chapter 10**: Getting unstuck, and ***Facing the Tiger* Chapter 11**: Grace under fire, prior to your next contact
- Complete the *Facing the Tiger* activity on page 130 on getting unstuck. You should provide a copy of **Tiger Activity Handout 9 — Getting Unstuck** for this activity (see Appendix 2.10).

Assessment

Administer the *Prostate Cancer Distress Screen* at the start of the session (see Appendix 3) to inform and guide the session content. If the man scores at 4 or above on the Distress Scale, check for the presence of anxiety and/or depression, and suicidal ideation, and manage accordingly.

Key Resources

This component relates to *Facing the Tiger* Chapter 10: Getting unstuck and *Facing the Tiger* Chapter 11: Grace under fire.

Chapter 10 outlines how to identify if you are ready for change and how to go about making changes.

- **Activity**: (*Facing the Tiger* page 130–133) Getting Unstuck. Use **Tiger Activity Handout 9 — Getting Unstuck** in Appendix 2.10.
- **Personal Stories:**

  Graeme talks about the setbacks and challenges he experienced from his prostate cancer diagnosis and after his partner died, and how he made a choice to open up to new experiences and reconnect with his community and his family in new ways.

Chapter 11 explores searching for meaning after a prostate cancer diagnosis and rebuilding your identity. There are no activities in this chapter.

- **Personal Stories:**

  Peter describes the challenges he took on after his prostate cancer and how this has influenced his life.

Flexible Component 8

Masculinity and Prostate Cancer

Introduction

Prostate cancer may present as a threat to a man's identity and sense of self in several ways. The first most obvious issue is the threat to sexuality that occurs as a consequence of treatment side effects such as erectile dysfunction, penile length, and sexual desire. More generally, if a man is receiving androgen deprivation therapy, he may also experience loss of muscle mass, central adiposity, breast swelling and hot flushes, which collectively may represent a feminising effect. But if one takes a broader view of masculinity, there are other potential impacts beyond these obvious issues around sexuality.

Research on masculinity in prostate cancer by the authors has identified five key domains of masculinity that are affected by prostate cancer:

1. **Optimistic Action**: an action-oriented approach to dealing with problems, for example, always looking for the good in a situation or taking action in the face of problems.
2. **Sexual Importance/Priority**: being able to have an erection and have sex.
3. **Family Responsibilities**: looking after your partner or family.

4. **Emotional Self-Reliance**: keeping your feelings to yourself or tending not to talk about your worries.
5. **Strength/Fitness**: being physically strong and an active person.

We approach masculinity from the perspective of internalised masculine beliefs or perceived masculine ideologies, adopting a nuanced approach that is contextualised and grounded in men's experiences.[75] These domains have been validated in a broad range of chronic diseases.[76]

Discussing with men the ways in which prostate cancer may affect feelings of masculinity or 'feeling like a man' provides a framework for them to deepen their awareness of what may be triggering their feelings of distress and from this develop strategies to rebuild or reinvent their sense of self.

Taking a strengths-based approach starts by helping men to better understand how their masculine values may influence their responses to illness. Awareness of when this is unhelpful (for example a risk taking or substance use response) and looking for ways to leverage off masculine values in a growth approach (for example connecting self-reliance to developing self-awareness and psychological flexibility) is likely more adaptive.[77,78]

Key Points

Introduce the concept of feelings of masculinity and their interaction with a diagnosis of prostate cancer by including the following points in your discussion.

- Masculinity for each man is individual, and understanding what values are important can help in understanding feelings of distress and why these feelings are difficult to sit with
- Masculine values can be sources of resilience. Becoming more self-aware and learning about self-management and applying these skills can support emotional self-reliance, and accessing optimistic action can be a motivation for change.

Discuss and generate possible actions to support important personal masculine values. This might include exercise training for strength/fitness, improving couple communication to strengthen emotional and sexual intimacy, increasing self-awareness of emotional triggers, and developing flexible strategies to manage distress.

Homework

- Provide the man with the **Masculinity in Health Inventory Worksheet** (see Appendix 2.10) explaining that there are no right or wrong answers and that the purpose is to help understand and reflect on how masculinity might be influencing his experience of prostate cancer.

Suggest that the man:

- Read or re-read ***Facing the Tiger* Chapter 2**, pages 19–22: Being a Man and Coping with Cancer prior to your next contact.
- If his masculinity concerns are around his sexual relationships, then ***Facing the Tiger* Chapter 4**: 'Me too!' On Loving Someone With Prostate Cancer and ***Facing the Tiger* Chapter 6:** Sex: What Now?, might be relevant.
- If he is more troubled by negative thoughts about himself as a man, consider ***Facing the Tiger* Chapter 7:** 'I think therefore I am!', ***Facing the Tiger* Chapter 10**: Getting Unstuck, and/or ***Facing the Tiger* Chapter 11**: Grace Under Fire.

Assessment

Administer the *Prostate Cancer Distress Screen* at the start of the session (see Appendix 3) to inform and guide the session content. If the man scores at 4 or above on the Distress Scale, check for the presence of anxiety and/or depression, and suicidal ideation, and manage accordingly.

Key Resources

Masculinity intersects across all aspects of a man's response to prostate cancer. This means that several of the *Facing the Tiger* chapters may be relevant depending on the man's key concerns. Refer to the Homework section above.

- **Masculinity in Health Inventory Worksheet** (Appendix 2.11).

Flexible Component 9

Prostate Cancer and Sexual Relationships

Introduction

Sexual relationships are an important part of many people's lives for reproduction, deepening and strengthening intimate relationships, pleasure and enjoyment, stress and tension release. Sexual intimacy can be self and life-affirming. Over the life course, sexual functioning can be negatively affected by many factors: relationship conflict, life stress, ageing, and psychological and physical illness or disturbance.

It is essential to be aware that medical and surgical treatments for prostate cancer frequently disrupt sexual function beyond the psychological distress of the cancer diagnosis. Side effects depend on the cancer treatment approach and can include erectile dysfunction, penile shortening, loss of libido, and loss of ejaculation.[79] These are not psychologically induced effects — they are a result of surgery or radiation therapy or the use of androgen deprivation therapy.

As such, managing these physical effects requires medical management from a specialist such as a urologist or sexual medical specialist and sexologist. In the short and often the long term, sexual activity will be changed after treatment. Coping with this change requires planning and communication between the man and his partner, preferably in advance of treatment as well as after treatment. The couple will need to try new approaches to sex and intimacy and be flexible about what sex looks like after a diagnosis of prostate cancer.

Sexual rehabilitation methods will be difficult for a couple to utilise effectively if their relationship is characterised by little or no emotional intimacy, a mismatch of goals about or interest in sex, and if the man and his partner are not comfortable talking about sex. The loss of spontaneity in sex after prostate cancer treatment, and the need often for invasive methods such as penile injections or using a vacuum pump, means adherence to sexual treatments after prostate cancer is often low over time,[80] with up to 80% of men discontinuing the use of medical interventions for erectile dysfunction following treatment.[81]

Furthermore, if a man and his partner have not been sexually active for years, one or both of them may have little interest in sexual rehabilitation. A female partner who is menopausal or post-menopausal may herself have low sexual desire and problems such as a dry vagina which make sexual activity difficult. She may have little interest in sex. Similarly, a partner who themselves has been experiencing health problems or declining health may have little interest in sexual activity. The diagnosis of prostate cancer can provide a pivot point for a couple to think about this aspect of their lives and make plans for change.

Key Points

It is important to ask about sexual changes and concerns to make sure the man has an avenue to discuss sexual rehabilitation goals and create an action plan for the future. Above all, the choices of the man and his partner need to be respected and supported.

Discussion about sexual rehabilitation should include the following points.

- Ask what sexual side effects the man's doctor has advised him are likely and explore the man's feelings and thoughts about these.
- Ensure the man has educational materials explaining side effects and possible sexual or penile rehabilitation approaches.
- It is generally accepted that the sooner a man commences penile rehabilitation, the better his long term outcome will be in terms of erections resuming.[82] After surgery erections can continue to improve up to two years after treatment.[83] Radiation therapy causes a slow, steady decline in erection strength from the start of treatment, stabilising around two years post-treatment.[84] Androgen deprivation therapy decreases a man's libido and ability

to achieve orgasm. Typically, the longer the duration of androgen deprivation therapy, the more persistent the effects will be, often persisting well after treatment ceases.[85]

- Encourage the man to discuss penile rehabilitation with his doctor. Some men may wish to delay sex until urinary incontinence has resolved. It is important to set goals and timelines for addressing sexual concerns.
- If the man has a partner, ask if they have discussed the sexual effects of treatment, what this means for them as a couple, and how they plan to approach this. If the man has not discussed this with his partner, encourage him to do so and practice or role-play ways he might bring the subject up. Coach the man through a problem-solving approach to recommencing sexual activity (see Flexible Component 5 — Problem Solving).
- The experience of erectile dysfunction is distressing even if the man is not sexually active. Having an erection for many men is part of 'being a man', and it is important to acknowledge this loss. Men can have similar feelings of loss about losing the ability to ejaculate.
- It is not uncommon for men to physically withdraw from their partner out of embarrassment or fear of not being able to perform sexually. This can lead the partner to feel unloved and for emotional intimacy to decline. Discuss with the man ways to maintain emotional intimacy and physical closeness without sex.

Homework

Suggest that the man:

- Read ***Facing the Tiger* Chapter 6**: Sex: What Now?, prior to your next contact.

Assessment

Administer the *Prostate Cancer Distress Screen* at the start of the session (see Appendix 3) to inform and guide the session content. If the man scores at 4 or above on the Distress Scale, check for the presence of anxiety and/or depression, and suicidal ideation, and manage accordingly.

Key Resources

This component relates to *Facing the Tiger* Chapter 6: Sex: What Now?

Chapter 6 outlines how sex might change after prostate cancer treatment, how to communicate these changes to a partner, and how to return to a normal sex life.

- **Activity**: (*Facing the Tiger* page 72) Getting sex back on track. Use **Tiger Activity Handout 10 — Getting Sex Back on Track** in Appendix 2.12.
- **Personal Stories:**

  Barbara and Geoff share how they approached getting their sex life back on track after treatment.

  Brad shares his experience as a young gay man diagnosed with prostate cancer and how he needed to rewire his thinking.

  Ian shares a story with a touch of humour and his advice to get on to it early.

Additional Resources

- **Flexible Component 4: Managing Relationships Under Stress** for communication strategies to maximise support and minimise the potential for withdrawal and/or conflict.
- **Flexible Component 5: Problem Solving** to address issues with sexual functioning by problem-solving.
- **Flexible Component 8: Masculinity and Prostate Cancer** on how sexual functioning affects feelings of masculinity.

Chapter 13

Flexible Component 10

Survivorship Care

Introduction

For most men, having prostate cancer leads to some changes in wellbeing. The type of changes and how long they persist will depend on the grade and stage of the man's cancer, the types of treatments received, and his overall health. Treatments for prostate cancer have dramatically improved and changed over the past two decades. Despite this, research shows that men and the doctors, nurses and allied health professionals who look after them report the experience of prostate cancer as being challenging, medically focused, and uncoordinated, with men's support needs often still not being adequately met.[29]

In all of this medical progress, change and evolution, the patient experience should be the central focus. Patient priorities and preferences should guide each step and each decision. Survivorship care recognises the physical, psychosocial, spiritual and economic impacts of cancer, which can be long-lasting, and addresses these so that the patient can achieve optimal quality of life.

Key Points

Introduce the concept of survivorship care by including the following points in your discussion.

- Any person who has had a cancer diagnosis is considered to be a survivor.
- Survivorship care means having a plan to look after your wellbeing now and for any changes that might happen in the future.
- There are six key areas of survivorship care to consider:
    - **Personal Agency:** This means taking control of what help you need and seeking support to manage your own health where you can. This does not mean going it alone. It means finding out who is there to help, what you can do yourself and what others can offer and being an active part of the team.
    - **Health Promotion and Advocacy**: Having accurate and up to date information about prostate cancer is important for you, your family and your community.
    - **Shared Management**: This means being an equal partner in your health care, sharing decision making with your health care team and sharing how you will tackle challenges as they arise. This includes informed decision making around testing and treatment, understanding and managing the physical and psychological effects of treatment and of the disease.
    - **Vigilance**: Your health care provider will manage surveillance from diagnosis and through life, including physical issues such as the control of the cancer and management of physical side effects and other illnesses that can occur as we age. This also includes checking on your emotional and social wellbeing.
    - **Care Coordination**: This is about your health care team working together to get you the best care possible in a 'right place at the right time' approach.
    - **Evidence-based Survivorship Interventions**: Your time and energy are valuable. Being evidence-based is about directing your time, energy and resources to strategies that have strong evidence to support their effectiveness. For example, there is excellent evidence for the benefits of exercise medicine. For overall wellness, good nutritional habits are important. Psychological support helps manage mood changes and the stress and anxiety associated with cancer. Sexual health support tailored to individual men in different age groups and with

different sexual orientations and relationships is also an area where good evidence exists about what works.

Key Procedures

Survivorship Care Planning

Provide the man with a copy of the *Survivorship Essentials Care Plan — My Personal Plan* (see Appendix 4 for download link) and include the following points in your discussion.

- A survivorship care plan is a summary of information about the man's diagnosis, treatment and ongoing care.
- The man may need a member of his Prostate Cancer healthcare team to assist him in completing the treatment plan part of the Survivorship Care Plan. Once this is completed, it is then important to keep it up to date.
- Suggest the man can take the plan with him to his health care appointments so that any care providers involved in his current and future care have a clear picture of his diagnosis and treatment.

Use the *Survivorship Essentials Care Plan* to discuss with the man what his priorities are for his wellbeing moving forward.

- Start by setting survivorship health and wellbeing goals and developing an action plan with a timeline. This sets the scene for a plan that is centred around **Personal Agency**. Targets for change need to be achievable adopting a flexible problem-solving approach as outlined in Flexible Component 5 — Problem Solving.
- Encourage the man to mobilise his social network as his support team and to consider reaching out to community supports and services around him. Suggest the man connects with his General Practitioner about his care plan as a central point of contact and his Specialist Prostate Cancer Nurse or Urology Nurse if he has access to this service. This is part of **Health Promotion and Advocacy**, **Shared Management**, and **Care Coordination** and helps in gaining mastery and control of the situation. Flexible Component 3: Making Decisions about Treatment can help prepare the man for conversations about his care.

- Check that he is clear about his clinical prostate cancer surveillance plan and check-up schedule and who has oversight of this. Talk to him about keeping a check on how he is managing from a psychological point of view and steps for checking on this, for example, using thought challenging strategies (Flexible Component 6). This is an important part of supporting **Vigilance** and being aware of and looking after your health physically as well as emotionally. Flexible Component 2: Stress Management and Wellbeing provides options for supporting physical and emotional wellbeing throughout his survivorship experience.
- Help the man seek clarity on who is the lead person coordinating his care and how he can contact them if needed. This helps with **Care Coordination**.
- Finally, discuss with the man what **Evidence-based Survivorship Interventions** are available to him and how he can locate services if new priorities or concerns emerge over time. You can build on the resources in each component of this manual, the supplementary health services listed in the *Survivorship Essentials Care Plan*, and resources listed in Appendix 1 to identify suitable local or readily accessible supports.

Homework

Suggest that the man:

- Read ***Facing the Tiger*** **Chapter 12**: Survivorship Care, prior to your next contact.

Assessment

Administer the *Prostate Cancer Distress Screen* at the start of the session (see Appendix 3) to inform and guide the session content. If the man scores at 4 or above on the Distress Scale, check for the presence of anxiety and/or depression, and suicidal ideation, and manage accordingly.

Key Resources

This component relates to *Facing the Tiger* Chapter 12: Survivorship Care.

Chapter 12 outlines the six key domains of survivorship care and how to apply them across the survivorship trajectory. There are no activities or personal stories in this chapter.

Additional Resources

- *Prostate Cancer Survivorship Care Plan* (See Appendix 4 for download link).

References

1. Watts S, Leydon G, Birch B, Prescott P, Lai L, Eardley S, et al. Depression and anxiety in prostate cancer: a systematic review and meta-analysis of prevalence rates. BMJ Open. 2014;4:e003901.
2. Dinkel A, Kornmayer M, Gschwend JE, Marten-Mittag B, Herschbach P, Herkommer K. Influence of family history on psychosocial distress and perceived need for treatment in prostate cancer survivors. Familial Cancer. 2014;13:481-8.
3. Sharp L, O'Leary E, Kinnear H, Gavin A, Drummond FJ. Cancer-related symptoms predict psychological wellbeing among prostate cancer survivors: results from the PiCTure study. Psycho-Oncology. 2016;25:282-91.
4. Smith DP, Supramaniam R, King MT, Ward J, Berry M, Armstrong BK. Age, health, and education determine supportive care needs of men younger than 70 years with prostate cancer. Journal of Clinical Oncology. 2007;25(18):2560-6.
5. Steginga SK, Occhipinti S, Dunn J, Gardiner RA, Heathcote P, Yaxley J. The supportive care needs of men with prostate cancer. Psycho-Oncology. 2001;10(1):66-75.
6. Hyde MK, Newton RU, Galvao DA, Gardiner RA, Occhipinti S, Lowe A, et al. Men's help-seeking in the first year after diagnosis of localised prostate cancer. European Journal of Cancer Care. 2017;26:e12497.
7. Smith DP, Calopedos R, Bang A, Yu XQ, Egger S, Chambers S, et al. Increased risk of suicide in New South Wales men with prostate cancer: Analysis of linked population-wide data. PLOS ONE. 2018;13(6):e0198679.
8. Watts S, Leydon G, Eyles C, Moore CM, Richardson A, Birch B, et al. A quantitative analysis of the prevalence of clinical depression and anxiety in patients with prostate cancer undergoing active surveillance. BMJ Open. 2015;5(5):e006674.
9. Guo Z, Gan S, Li Y, Gu C, Xiang S, Zhou J, et al. Incidence and risk factors of suicide after a prostate cancer diagnosis: a meta-analysis of observational studies. Prostate Cancer and Prostatic Diseases. 2018;21:499–508.
10. Bill-Axelson A, Garmo H, Lambe M, Bratt O, Adolfsson J, Nyberg U, et al. Suicide risk in men with prostate-specific antigen-detected early prostate cancer: a nationwide population-based cohort study from PCBaSe

Sweden. European Urology. 2010;57(3):390-5.

11. Carlsson S, Sandin F, Fall K, Lambe M, Adolfsson J, Stattin P, et al. Risk of suicide in men with low-risk prostate cancer. European Journal of Cancer. 2013;49(7):1588-99.
12. Fang F, Keating NL, Mucci LA, Adami H, Stampfer MJ, Valdimarsdottir U, et al. Immediate Risk of Suicide and Cardiovascular Death After a Prostate Cancer Diagnosis: Cohort Study in the United States. Journal of the National Cancer Institute. 2010;102(5).
13. Orom H, Biddle C, Underwood W, 3rd, Nelson CJ. Worse Urinary, Sexual and Bowel Function Cause Emotional Distress and Vice Versa in Men Treated for Prostate Cancer. Journal of Urology. 2018;199(6):1464-9.
14. Nguyen C, Lairson DR, Swartz MD, Du XL. Risks of Major Long-Term Side Effects Associated with Androgen-Deprivation Therapy in Men with Prostate Cancer. Pharmacotherapy. 2018;38(10):999-1009.
15. Rhee H, Gunter JH, Heathcote P, Ho K, Stricker P, Corcoran NM, et al. Adverse effects of androgen-deprivation therapy in prostate cancer and their management. BJU International. 2015;115 Suppl 5:3-13.
16. Smith DP, King MT, Egger S, Berry MP, Stricker PD, Cozzi P, et al. Quality of life three years after diagnosis of localised prostate cancer: population based cohort study. BMJ: British Medical Journal. 2009;339:b4817.
17. Paterson C, Primeau C, Howard N, Xiberras P, Pillay B, Crowe H. Experiences of Unmet Need and Access to Supportive Care for Men Receiving Androgen Deprivation Therapy for Prostate Cancer: A Bi-national Study. Seminars in Oncology Nursing. 2020;36(4):151049.
18. Thomas HR, Chen M-H, D'Amico AV, Bennett CL, Kattan MW, Sartor O, et al. Association Between Androgen Deprivation Therapy and Patient-reported Depression in Men With Recurrent Prostate Cancer. Clinical Genitourinary Cancer. 2018;16(4):313-7.
19. Mazariego CG, Juraskova I, Campbell R, Smith DP. Long-term unmet supportive care needs of prostate cancer survivors: 15-year follow-up from the NSW Prostate Cancer Care and Outcomes Study. Supportive Care in Cancer. 2020 Nov;28(11):5511-5520.
20. Crawford-Williams F, March S, Goodwin BC, Ralph N, Galvão DA, Newton RU, et al. Interventions for prostate cancer survivorship: A systematic review of reviews. Psycho-Oncology. 2018;27(10):2339-48.
21. Chambers SK, Hyde MK, Smith DP, Hughes S, Yuill S, Egger S, et al. New Challenges in Psycho-Oncology Research III: A systematic review of psychological interventions for prostate cancer survivors and their partners: clinical and research implications. Psycho-Oncology. 2017;26(7):873-913.

22. Chambers SK, Heathcote P. The psychological toll of prostate cancer. Nature Reviews Urology. 2018;15:733–4.

23. Surbone A, Tralongo P. Categorization of Cancer Survivors: Why We Need. Journal of Clinical Oncology. 2016;34(28):3372-4.

24. Narayan V, Harrison M, Cheng H, Kenfield S, Aggarwal R, Kwon D, et al. Improving research for prostate cancer survivorship: A statement from the Survivorship Research in Prostate Cancer (SuRECaP) working group. Urologic Oncology. 2020;38(3):83-93.

25. Feuerstein M. Defining cancer survivorship. Journal of Cancer Survivorship 2007;1(1):5-7.

26. National Cancer Institute. Office of Cancer Survivorship 2019. Available from: https://cancercontrol.cancer.gov/ocs/.

27. Skolarus TA, Wolf AMD, Erb NL, Brooks DD, Rivers BM, Underwood III W, et al. American Cancer Society prostate cancer survivorship care guidelines. CA: A Cancer Journal for Clinicians. 2014;64(4):225-49.

28. Sanft T, Denlinger CS, Armenian S, Baker KS, Broderick G, Demark-Wahnefried W, et al. NCCN Guidelines Insights: Survivorship, Version 2.2019. Journal of the National Comprehensive Cancer Network. 2019;17(7):784-94.

29. Dunn J, Ralph N, Green A, Frydenberg M, Chambers S. Contemporary consumer perspectives on prostate cancer survivorship: Fifty voices. Psycho-Oncology. 2019 Mar;29(3):557-563.

30. Dunn J, Green A, Ralph N, Newton R, Kneebone A, Frydenberg M, et al. Prostate Cancer Survivorship Essentials Framework: Guidelines for Practitioners. BJU International. 2020; https://doi.org/10.1111/bju.15159.

31. Bennett-Levy J, Richards DA, Farrand P. Low intensity CBT interventions: A revolution in mental health care. Oxford guide to low intensity CBT interventions. Oxford guides in cognitive behavioural therapy. New York, NY, US: Oxford University Press; 2010. p. 3-18.

32. Holland J, Watson M, Dunn J. The IPOS new International Standard of Quality Cancer Care: integrating the psychosocial domain into routine care. Psycho-Oncology. 2011;20(7):677-80.

33. Hutchison SD, Steginga SK, Dunn J. The tiered model of psychosocial intervention in cancer: a community based approach. Psycho-Oncology. 2006;15(6):541-6.

34. Carey T. Will you follow while they lead? Introducing a patient-led approach to low intensity CBT interventions. In: Bennett-Levy J, et al., editor. Oxford Guide to Low Intensity CBT Interventions. New York, NY, US: Oxford University Press; 2010. p. 331-8.

35. Dunn J, Steginga SK, Rosoman N, Millichap D. A Review of Peer Support in the Context of Cancer. Journal of Psychosocial Oncology. 2003;21(2):55-67.

36. Cohen S, Wills TA. Stress, social support, and the buffering hypothesis. Psychological Bulletin. 1985;98(2):310-57.

37. Taylor SE. Social Support. In: Friedman H, editor. The Oxford Handbook of Health Psychology. New York: Oxford University Press; 2011. p. 189-214.

38. Cutrona CE, Russell DW. Type of social support and specific stress: Toward a theory of optimal matching. Social support: An interactional view. Wiley series on personality processes. Oxford, England: John Wiley & Sons; 1990. p. 319-66.

39. Lazarus RS, Folkman S. Stress, Appraisal, and Coping. New York: Springer; 1984.

40. Folkman S. Positive psychological states and coping with severe stress. Soc ial Science & Medicine 1997;45(8):1207-21.

41. Folkman S. The case for positive emotions in the stress process. Anxiety, Stress, & Coping. 2008;21(1):3-14.

42. Biggs A, Brough P, Drummond S. Lazarus and Folkman's psychological stress and coping theory. The handbook of stress and health: A guide to research and practice. Hoboken, NJ, US: Wiley Blackwell; 2017. p. 351-64.

43. Ralph N, Ng SK, Zajdlewicz L, Lepore SJ, Heathcote P, Kneebone A, et al. Ten-year quality of life outcomes in men with prostate cancer. Psycho-Oncology. 2020;29(2):444-9.

44. Nezu AM, Nezu CM, Friedman SH, Faddis S, Houts PS. Helping cancer patients cope: A problem-solving approach. Washington, DC, US: American Psychological Association; 1998.

45. Hayes SC. A Liberated Mind: How to Pivot Toward What Matters: Penguin Publishing Group; 2019.

46. Horvath AO, Luborsky L. The role of the therapeutic alliance in psychotherapy. Journal of Consulting and Clinical Psychology. 1993;61(4):561-73.

47. Ackerman SJ, Hilsenroth MJ. A review of therapist characteristics and techniques positively impacting the therapeutic alliance. Clinical Psychology Review. 2003;23(1):1-33.

48. Ell KO, Mantell JE, Hamovitch MB, Nishimoto RH. Social Support, Sense of Control, and Coping Among Patients with Breast, Lung, or Colorectal Cancer. Journal of Psychosocial Oncology. 1989;7(3):63-89.

49. Ardito RB, Rabellino D. Therapeutic alliance and outcome of psychotherapy: historical excursus, measurements, and prospects for research.

Frontiers in Psychology. 2011;2:270-.

50. Baier AL, Kline AC, Feeny NC. Therapeutic alliance as a mediator of change: A systematic review and evaluation of research. Clinical Psychology Review. 2020;82:101921.
51. Chambers SK, Zajdlewicz L, Youlden DR, Holland JC, Dunn J. The validity of the distress thermometer in prostate cancer populations. Psycho-Oncology. 2014;23(2):195-203.
52. Holland J, Watson M, Dunn J. The IPOS New International Standard of Quality Cancer Care: integrating the psychosocial domain into routine care. Psycho-Oncology. 2011;20(7):677-80.
53. Vodermaier A, Linden W, Siu C. Screening for emotional distress in cancer patients: a systematic review of assessment instruments. Journal of the National Cancer Institute. 2009;101(21):1464-88.
54. Prostate Cancer Foundation of Australia and University of Southern Queensland. My Personal Plan: A survivorship care plan for men with prostate cancer. ISBN 978-0-6452955-0-4. 2021.
55. Jacobsen PB, Donovan KA, Trask PC, Fleishman SB, Zabora J, Baker F, et al. Screening for psychologic distress in ambulatory cancer patients. Cancer. 2005;103(7):1494-502.
56. Bevans M, Wehrlen L, Prachenko O, Soeken K, Zabora J, Wallen GR. Distress screening in allogeneic hematopoietic stem cell (HSCT) caregivers and patients. Psycho-Oncology. 2011;20(6):615-22.
57. Bidstrup PE, Mertz BG, Dalton SO, Deltour I, Kroman N, Kehlet H, et al. Accuracy of the Danish version of the 'distress thermometer'. Psycho-Oncology. 2012;21(4):436-43.
58. Craike MJ, Livingston PM, Warne C. Sensitivity and specificity of the distress impact thermometer for the detection of psychological distress among CRC survivors. Journal of Psychosocial Oncology. 2011;29(3):231-41.
59. Gunnarsdottir S, Thorvaldsdottir G, Fridriksdottir N, Bjarnason B, Sigurdsson F, Skulason B, et al. The psychometric properties of the Icelandic version of the Distress Thermometer and Problem List. Psycho-Oncology. 2012;21(7):730-6.
60. Hawkes AL, Hughes KL, Hutchison SD, Chambers SK. Feasibility of brief psychological distress screening by a community-based telephone helpline for cancer patients and carers. BMC Cancer. 2010;10(1):14.
61. Hegel MT, Collins ED, Kearing S, Gillock KL, Moore CP, Ahles TA. Sensitivity and specificity of the Distress Thermometer for depression in newly diagnosed breast cancer patients. Psycho-Oncology. 2008;17(6):556-60.

62. Roerink SH, de Ridder M, Prins J, Huijbers A, de Wilt HJ, Marres H, et al. High level of distress in long-term survivors of thyroid carcinoma: Results of rapid screening using the distress thermometer. Acta Oncologica. 2013;52(1):128-37.

63. Shim EJ, Shin YW, Jeon HJ, Hahm BJ. Distress and its correlates in Korean cancer patients: pilot use of the distress thermometer and the problem list. Psycho-Oncology. 2008;17(6):548-55.

64. Tuinman MA, Gazendam-Donofrio SM, Hoekstra-Weebers JE. Screening and referral for psychosocial distress in oncologic practice. Cancer. 2008;113(4):870-8.

65. Kroenke K, Spitzer RL, Williams JB. The PHQ-9: validity of a brief depression severity measure. Journal of General Internal Medicine. 2001;16(9):606-13.

66. Spitzer RL, Kroenke K, Williams JB, Löwe B. A brief measure for assessing generalized anxiety disorder: the GAD-7. Archives of Internal Medicine. 2006;166(10):1092-7.

67. Fisher K, Seidler ZE, King K, Oliffe JL, Rice SM. Men's anxiety: A systematic review. Journal of Affective Disorders. 2021;295:688-702.

68. Cormie P, Atkinson M, Bucci L, Cust A, Eakin E, Hayes S, et al. Clinical Oncology Society of Australia position statement on exercise in cancer care. Medical Journal of Australia. 2018;209(4):184-7.

69. Campbell KL, Winters-Stone KM, Wiskemann J, May AM, Schwartz AL, Courneya KS, et al. Exercise Guidelines for Cancer Survivors: Consensus Statement from International Multidisciplinary Roundtable. Medicine & Science in Sports & Exercise. 2019;51(11).

70. Hayes SC, Newton RU, Spence RR, Galvão DA. The Exercise and Sports Science Australia position statement: Exercise medicine in cancer management. Journal of Science and Medicine in Sport. 2019;22(11):1175-99.

71. Godin G. The Godin-Shephard Leisure-Time Physical Activity Questionnaire. The Health & Fitness Journal of Canada. 2011;4(1):18-22.

72. Galvão DA, Taaffe DR, Spry N, Cormie P, Joseph D, Chambers SK, et al. Exercise Preserves Physical Function in Prostate Cancer Patients with Bone Metastases. Medicine & Science in Sports & Exercise. 2018;50(3):393-9.

73. The Ottawa Hospital Research Institute and University of Ottawa. Ottawa Personal Decision Guide 2015. Available from: https://decisionaid.ohri.ca/docs/das/OPDG.pdf.

74. Steven C. Hayes. My ACT Tool Kit 2021. Available from: https://steven-

chayes.com/my-act-toolkit/.

75. Chambers SK, Hyde MK, Oliffe JL, Zajdlewicz L, Lowe A, Wootten AC, et al. Measuring Masculinity in the Context of Chronic Disease. Psychology of Men & Masculinity. 2016;17(3):228-42.
76. Occhipinti S, Laurie K, Hyde MK, Martin S, Oliffe J, Wittert G, et al. Measuring Masculinity in Men With Chronic Disease. American Journal of Men's Health. 2019;13(4):1557988319859706.
77. Rice SM, Kealy D, Ogrodniczuk JS, Seidler ZE, Denehy L, Oliffe JL. The Cost of Bottling It Up: Emotion Suppression as a Mediator in the Relationship Between Anger and Depression Among Men with Prostate Cancer. Cancer Management and Research. 2020;12:1039-46.
78. Rice SM, Kealy D, Ogrodniczuk JS, Seidler ZE, Montaner G, Chambers S, et al. The Anxiety Depression Pathway Among Men Following a Prostate Cancer Diagnosis: Cross-Sectional Interactions Between Anger Responses and Loneliness. The World Journal of Men's Health. 2021;15(3):15579883211023699.
79. Hyun JS. Prostate cancer and sexual function. The World Journal of Men's Health. 2012;30(2):99-107.
80. Albaugh J, Adamic B, Chang C, Kirwen N, Aizen J. Adherence and barriers to penile rehabilitation over 2 years following radical prostatectomy. BMC Urology. 2019;19(1):89.
81. Schover LR, Fouladi RT, Warneke CL, Neese L, Klein EA, Zippe C, et al. Defining sexual outcomes after treatment for localized prostate carcinoma. Cancer. 2002;95(8):1773-85.
82. Chung E, Gillman M. Prostate cancer survivorship: a review of erectile dysfunction and penile rehabilitation after prostate cancer therapy. Medical Journal of Australia. 2014;200(10):582-5.
83. Emanu JC, Avildsen IK, Nelson CJ. Erectile dysfunction after radical prostatectomy: prevalence, medical treatments, and psychosocial interventions. Current Opinion in Supportive and Palliative Care. 2016;10(1):102-7.
84. van der Wielen GJ, Mulhall JP, Incrocci L. Erectile dysfunction after radiotherapy for prostate cancer and radiation dose to the penile structures: A critical review. Radiotherapy and Oncology. 2007;84(2):107-13.
85. Grossmann M, Zajac JD. Management of side effects of androgen deprivation therapy. Endocrinology and Metabolism Clinics of North America. 2011;40(3):655-71, x.

Appendix

Resources

This is a brief list of books, websites and organisations that can be helpful for men with prostate cancer and their partners. Contact details were accurate at time of printing. For medical or treatment questions your doctor is the best first point of call for advice that is personalised to your situation.

Helpful Information

Facing Prostate Cancer

The Prostate Playbook: Keep It. Healthy. Craig Allingham. Redsok Publications, Australia. 2019. ISBN 978098706670.

Gay and Bisexual Men Living with Prostate Cancer From Diagnosis to Recovery. Edited by Jane Ussher, Janette Perz, and B. R. Simon Rosser. Harrington Park Press, LLC, New York. 2018. ISBN 9781939594259. Also available as an ebook.

Sex and Sexuality

Saving Your Sex Life: A Guide for Men with Prostate Cancer. John P. Mulhall. Hilton Publishing, Bethesda, MD. 2010. ISBN 9780980064964. Also available as an ebook on Kindle.

After Prostate Cancer: A What-comes-next guide to a safe and informed recovery. Arnold Melman MD and Rosemary E. Newnham. Oxford University Press, New York. 2011. ISBN 9780195399660. Also available as an ebook on Kindle.

A Gay Man's Guide to Prostate Cancer. Gerald Perlman and Jack Drescher. Haworth Medical Press, United States. 2005. ISBN 9781560235521.

www.renewintimacy.org The Center for Intimacy after Cancer Therapy, Inc. is a non-profit organisation dedicated to helping couples renew their intimacy after cancer. Founders and Co-Executive Directors: Ralph and Barbara Alterowitz.

www.thepenisproject.org The Penis Project podcast is hosted by Sexologist and Nurse Practitioner, Melissa Hadley Barrett and Physiotherapist Dr Jo Milios who talk to real men and the experts about men's private parts.

Urinary Problems

Conquering Incontinence: A New and Physical Approach to a Freer Lifestyle Exercise. Peter Dornan. Allen & Unwin, Australia 2003. ISBN 9781741141443. Also available as an ebook on Kindle.

Prostate Recovery MAP: Men's Action Plan. Craig Allingham. Redsok, Australia. 2013. ISBN 9780987076656.

Mindfulness and Meditation

Happy For No Good Reason: A meditators guide. Swami Shankarananda. Motilal Banasidass, India. 2004. ISBN 9788120820050. Also available as an ebook on Kindle.

Full Catastrophe Living (Revised Edition): Using the Wisdom of Your Body and Mind to Face Stress, Pain, and Illness. Jon Kabat-Zinn. Delta Publishing, United Kingdom. 2013. ISBN 9780345536938. Also available as an ebook on Kindle.

Complementary Medicine

Promoting Wellness for Prostate Cancer Patients: A guide for men and their families. Fourth Edition. Mark A Moyad. Spry Publishing LLC, United States. 2013. ISBN 9781938170034.

Wellbeing

What Women (and Their Men) Need to Know About Prostate Cancer. Irena Madjar in collaboration with Gail Tingle. Prostate Survival Alliance Inc., Australia. 2008. ISBN 9780646482965.

Advice about Exercise

www.essa.org.au Exercise and Sports Science Australia (ESSA) — provide details of registered exercise professionals with University qualifications who are able to conduct exercise training with people who have had cancer or other chronic illnesses. The ESSA website has a section in their main page on How to

Find an Accredited Exercise Physiologist (AEP) and you can select 'cancer' as a speciality: https://www.essa.org.au/find-aep.

www.acsm.org American College of Sports Medicine (ACSM) provides a similar service.

www.bases.org.uk The British Association of Sport and Exercise Sciences, BASES provides a similar service in the United Kingdom.

Sources of Information and Support

Australia

www.pcfa.org.au/support To contact a prostate cancer support group in your local area look up the *Prostate Cancer Foundation of Australia* website or call freecall: 1800 220 099. The Prostate Cancer Foundation of Australia (PCFA) is a broad-based community organisation and the peak national body for prostate cancer in Australia dedicated to reducing the impact of prostate cancer on Australian men, their partners, families and the wider community. PCFA can provide you with written information about prostate cancer and its treatment and can connect you to relevant services, including:

- The PCFA Prostate Cancer Telenursing Support Service: https://www.prostate.org.au/prostate-cancer-specialist-telenursing-service/
- Telephone-based peer support via PCFA Mates Connect Program: https://www.prostate.org.au/support/matesconnect-phone-based-peer-support/

The *Cancer Council Helpline* is a free, confidential telephone information and support service run by Cancer Councils in each state and territory in Australia. Specially trained staff are available to answer questions about cancer and provide support. Call 13 11 20 (local call cost from anywhere in Australia but mobile calls charged at mobile rates), open between 9am and 5pm, Monday to Friday, however some states have extended hours.

New Zealand

www.prostate.org.nz/support-groups To contact a prostate cancer support group in your local area look up the *Prostate Cancer Foundation of New Zealand* website or call 0800 477 678. The Prostate Cancer Foundation of New Zealand aims to help those recently diagnosed with prostate cancer, and survivors of prostate cancer, to lead productive and full lives through shared counselling and discussions.

www.cancernz.org.nz The *Cancer Society of New Zealand* has a free Cancer Information Helpline, 0800 CANCER (226 237), which supplies booklets, information sheets and other information resources which can also be downloaded directly from their website.

North America

www.ustoo.org *Us TOO International Prostate Cancer Education and Support Network* is a non-profit, grassroots organisation that provides support for prostate cancer patients, survivors, their spouses and partners and families. More details can be found on their website. They have a toll free line to link for patients and concerned others to resources regarding diagnosis, treatment options and support systems and phone support from a prostate cancer survivor. Call 1-800-80-UsTOO (1-800-808-7866), open between 9am and 5pm, Monday to Friday, Central Time.

http://malecare.org *Malecare* develops practical, life-enhancing men's health programs and has a focus on gay and bisexual men's survivorship. Malecare runs a series of workshops and Prostate Cancer Support groups throughout the United States in areas of newly diagnosed cancer support groups, advanced prostate cancer, men diagnosed under age 50 and gay cancer survivor support.

Canada

www.prostatecancer.ca In early 2020, *Prostate Cancer Canada* amalgamated with the *Canadian Cancer Society*. As well as connecting you to support groups the website also hosts a series of Expert Angle webinars, which cover many different prostate cancer related topics.

United Kingdom

www.tackleprostate.org The *National Federation of Prostate Cancer Support Groups* can connect you to a support group through their free Helpline on 0800 035 5302 or via their website.

https://prostatecanceruk.org *Prostate Cancer UK* provides a free hotline and live website chat run by specialist nurses, which can be accessed via their website or by calling 0800 074 8383. There are also options for local and online support groups, a dedicated online community, and one-to-one support provided by trained volunteers.

www.prostatescotland.org.uk *Prostate Scotland* is a Scottish charity set up to provide information, advice and help on prostate cancer. They can connect you to support groups across the country. They also provide a range of information.

Europe

www.europa-uomo.org *Europa Uomo* (Italian for Europe man) is a European advocacy movement representing 27 prostate patients' groups in countries across Europe. Details of member organisations in each country, and in the countries' language, can be found on their website.

Survivorship

Dunn J, Casey C, Sandoe D, Hyde MK, Cheron-Sauer M-C, Lowe A, Oliffe J & Chambers SK. ***Advocacy, Support and Survivorship in Prostate Cancer.*** (2018) European Journal of Cancer Care. 27(2) e12644. doi: 10.1111/ecc.12644 — This article describes the development of the prostate cancer support network in Australia. Direct open access link: **https://onlinelibrary.wiley.com/doi/full/10.1111/ecc.12644**

Dunn J, Green A, Ralph N, Newton R, Kneebone A, Frydenberg M, Chambers SK. ***Prostate Cancer Survivorship Essentials Framework: Guidelines for Practitioners*** (2020). British Journal of Urology International. https://doi.org/10.1111/bju.15159. — This paper further describes the framework for prostate cancer survivorship from Facing the Tiger Chapter 12, and was developed by clinical and community groups in Australia and New Zealand. Direct open access link: **https://bjuijournals.onlinelibrary.wiley.com/doi/10.1111/bju.15159**

www.cancer.net/survivorship/follow-care-after-cancer treatment/ asco-cancer-treatment-and-survivorship-care-plans The *American Society of Clinical Oncology* has developed two forms to help people diagnosed with cancer keep track of the treatment they received and medical care they may need in the future: a Cancer Treatment Plan and a Survivorship Care Plan.

www.petermac.org/sites/default/files/media-uploads/ACSC_Factsheet_SurvivorshipCarePlans.pdf This is an Australian version developed by the *Australian Cancer Survivorship Centre.*

www.prostate.org.au/awareness/for-healthcare-professionals/ screening-for-distress The Prostate Cancer Foundation of Australia has a *Distress Screening Tool* for health professionals to use with men to assess their level of distress and identify key problems. The tool is to help your health care provider ensure that your emotional and psychological wellbeing needs are being addressed. A score of 4 or more on the Distress Thermometer needs a conversation with your doctor or nurse about how you are tracking.

www.servicesaustralia.gov.au/individuals/services/centrelink/disability-support-pension/what-resources-are-available/disability-employment-services/work-assist Work Assist is an Australian government service that can help to redesign your job so you can keep working, change your workplace so you can continue to work, or get specialised equipment to help you do your job.

Other Useful Websites

www.prostatenet.com *The Prostate Net* is an international organisation that uses a matrix of informational techniques (web site, 800#, email and personal team counsellors, public forums, newsletters and community disease interventions) to address disease risk awareness and early disease detection.

Appendix 2

Client Handouts

Clients handouts required for each session are listed below with their Appendix number and title. You are free to photocopy the handouts from the following pages (they will reproduce best at a magnification of 125%) or use the QR code link below to download a PDF document containing all Appendix 2 handouts. An email address is all that is required to immediately begin the download.

https://sowl.co/3ntgo

Appendix 2.1	Tiger Activity Handout 1Awareness of Responses to Stress and Coping Strategies
Appendix 2.2	Tiger Activity Handout 2 Goal Setting
Appendix 2.3	Tiger Relaxation Handout
Appendix 2.4	Tiger Activity Handout 3 Mindfulness Focussing
Appendix 2.5	Tiger Activity Handout 4 Goal Setting to De-stress
Appendix 2.6	Tiger Activity Handout 5 Treatment Decision Making
Appendix 2.7	Tiger Activity Handout 6 Problem Solving
Appendix 2.8	Tiger Activity Handout 7 Automatic Thinking
Appendix 2.9	Tiger Activity Handout 8 Identifying Patterns of Thinking
Appendix 2.10	Tiger Activity Handout 9 Getting Unstuck
Appendix 2.11	Worksheet: Masculinity in Health Inventory
Appendix 2.12	Tiger Activity Handout 10 Getting Sex Back on Track

Tiger Activity Handout 1

Awareness of Responses to Stress and Coping Strategies

(See *Facing the Tiger* Chapter 1, page 6.)

STEP 1: As a first step think about how you felt when you first found out about the cancer and see if you can recall the thoughts that ran through your mind.

- Did you have one strong worry, or a stream of concerns that rapidly replaced each other?
- Was there one strong emotion you felt? How did your body respond physically?
- What was your first coping reaction?
- Did you look for a cave for comfort or did you come out fighting?

Taking some time to sit with these feelings and thoughts will help you to increase your awareness of what the diagnosis means to you. This might be uncomfortable, but awareness is the first step to understanding your response, your strengths, and your challenge points.

STEP 2: Next, fill in examples in each circle below of what sort of thoughts, emotions, physical reactions and actions you remember feeling and doing.

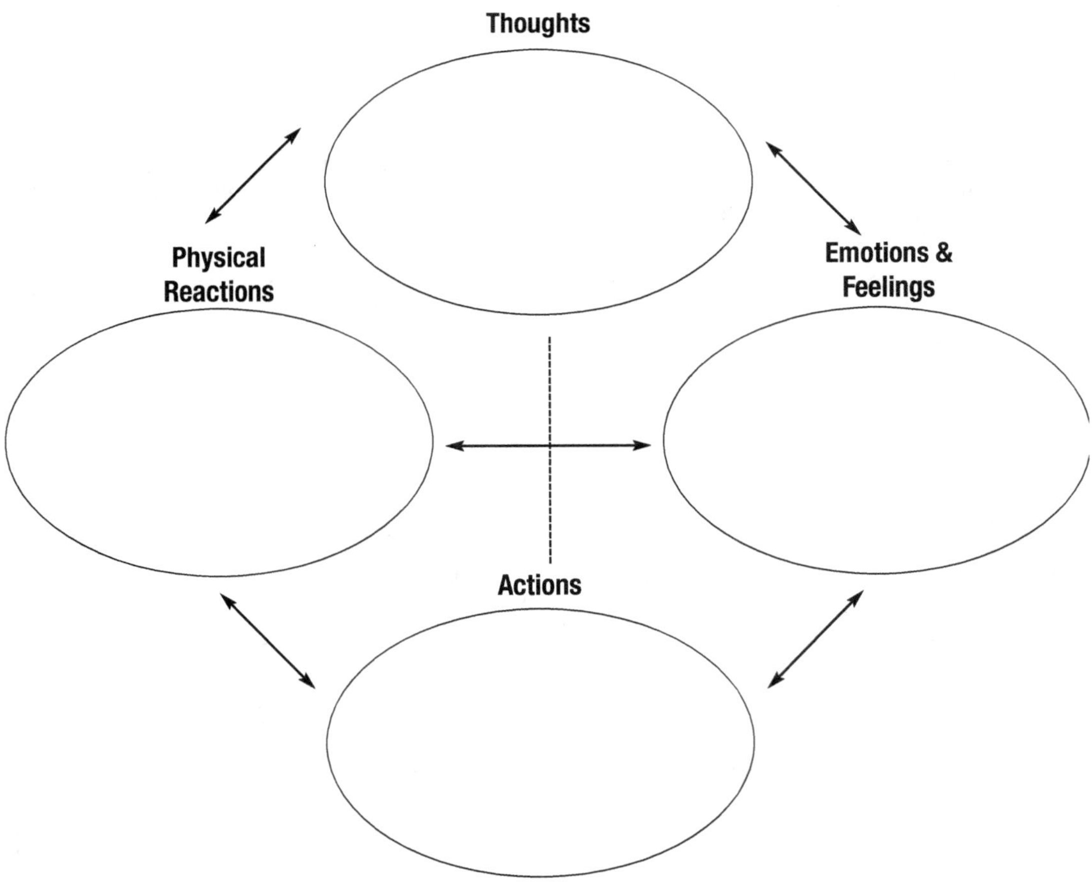

STEP 3: What actions did you take that were helpful?

What did not work so well?

Now think back to a different example in your life when you have had a difficult time, perhaps a job loss, serious illness in someone you cared for, the death of a loved one, the end of a relationship. Were your feelings then similar to now, or different?

Do you have a typical way of coping with stress, and how well does this serve you?

Goal Setting

(See *Facing the Tiger* Chapter 2, page 24.)

For most men at whatever stage of life, a prostate cancer diagnosis threatens their goals and hopes. How has cancer affected your goals and future hopes? Write these down in your own dedicated notebook or in the space below.

____

____

____

Perhaps your goals have changed since the cancer diagnosis and other things have become more important. Looking at your list, which of these matters most to you right now?

____

____

____

Each of your goals will have a different timeline; some might be things you would like to achieve in the short- or medium-term; some might be long-term goals. You might set goals that are about how you are coping with the cancer; or about your relationships and how you would like them to be or to develop.

As an example, a short-term goal might be to learn some quick and easy stress reduction strategies, such as deep breathing exercises and a low intensity walking program. As you do this, you can map your overall well-being so you can be encouraged by the gains you make.

A plan to improve your sexual life might start with short-term goals about pleasant couple activities (such as seeing a movie or going for a dinner 'date') and intimacy, and sensual pleasure, with a medium-term goal to have full sexual intercourse.

Long-term goals might be to complete treatment and then go on a long-awaited holiday (best not to wait for 'one day') or to take on a personal physical or mental challenge. You might have long-term life goals you would like to work towards.

What would you like life to look like for you in six or twelve months?

____

____

____

____

Next, start to list what steps you need to take to achieve these goals?

Finally, who can help you with this? Jot down the names of people in your life you could enlist to support, help or encourage you to reach these goals. Talk to someone you trust or who is close to you about your most hoped for goals. This will help you further clarify and confirm your next steps.

Every month or so check back with your list and see how you are going. It is perfectly fine if your list changes, or if new goals come up. The main point of this activity is that you have a sense of direction and that you notice when you achieve goals, and then give yourself a pat on the back!

Now for your toolbox! How do you usually cope with difficulties?

What is your main preference and how well does that work for you?

____

Think about a time when you have coped well with a personal challenge and felt very positive about the outcome. How would you describe your approach then?

Now think about a time when you were faced with a personal challenge and it did not go so well. How could you have approached this problem differently?

Tiger Relaxation Handout

FACING THE TIGER

Learning to Relax — Practice makes Perfect

Find a private quiet place where you won't be disturbed. Make sure you are wearing relaxed clothes. Sit comfortably and focus for a few minutes on being aware of your breathing, then do the following:

- Notice how your breath moves in and out of your nose and chest, and how your chest muscles contract and relax as you breathe.
- Listen to the sound of your breath as you breathe in and out.
- Be aware of your posture and how your shoulders sit as you breathe. If your shoulders are tight and hunched drop them down on your out-breath.
- Next, count slowly to four in every in and out-breath you take. Focus your mind on the count, and breathe in a slow and relaxed and comfortable way in time to the count. Do this for several minutes as your body gets used to slow and controlled breathing.
- Now stop and notice how you feel.

This is a quick and easy de-stress strategy that can be easily applied to good effect when stuck in traffic, waiting in a doctor's office for a check-up, or at night just before going to sleep to relax yourself down. It can be extended by adding in at the end a couple of extra breaths where you hold between breathes for a count of two.

You can also add visualisation or imagery by focussing your mind on a safe and relaxing scenario or image, once your breathing has slowed down. This might mean building a picture in your mind of a relaxing place and activity, such as swimming in the sea or walking in a forest, and imagining the colours and sounds and physical sensations he would experience if your were there.

This is a quick, easy and portable strategy for use in any situation that triggers tension.

Tiger Activity Handout 3

Mindfulness Focussing

(See *Facing the Tiger* Chapter 8, pages 96–97.)

Find a place in the garden or a quiet room where you can sit comfortably and uninterrupted for about ten minutes. The goal of this exercise is to stop and become aware of your physical location and your surroundings sense-by-sense. Before you start, check your watch.

First, become aware of how you feel now that you have stopped what you were doing. What thoughts — or echoes of thoughts — have you carried with you into this moment and what feelings are here now? Perhaps scan your body and notice if there are any points of tightness or tension in your body. Next — deliberately gather your attention and redirect it to the feeling of your breath as it enters, and then again, as it leaves your body. Do this for several breaths — almost as if you are dropping anchor into this moment using your breath. Now expand your awareness around your breath and begin to notice how you feel physically in this space. Are you cool or warm? Feel the bottom of your feet and how your feet feel against the ground. Are you sitting firmly? How does your backside feel against the chair? Your back?

Listen to the sounds around you. What can you hear in the background? Road noise? Birds? The sound of your breathing? Choose one sound and try to notice the details of the sound — the volume, the pitch, the gaps between the sounds. Notice if your mind starts to tell you stories about what you can hear, and, as best you can bring your mind back to focus on the details of the sounds themselves.

Now look around you and find a visual point on which to focus. It might be a plant leaf or a photograph on the wall. Closely notice the details of this point. Notice the shades of colour, the texture, the shape — how the sun falls on this spot. Maintain this focus as long as you can and try and notice the details that you might not have seen before.

Now, check your watch again. How long were you able to keep this up for? Three minutes? Five? It can be surprisingly hard to stop for ten minutes and become aware of our surroundings. How did you feel while you were doing this exercise? What was the state of your mind? Did you feel frustrated at being still or did you feel a sense of calm?

Goal Setting to De-stress

(See *Facing the Tiger* Chapter 8, page 100.)

STEP 1: Think about how you feel most of the time, do you think you have room for improvement in the way you look after yourself? Use the checklist below as a start and prioritise which of these things you would most like to work on.

- ☐ Exercising more
- ☐ Feeing calmer
- ☐ Reducing my weight
- ☐ Feeling physically stronger
- ☐ Any other ways?

STEP 2: The next step is to draw up a plan of attack. Be clear about your goals first and the short and medium-term milestones you want to reach, and when you expect to get there.

List the steps you will need to take to move towards these milestones, who and what you need to help you achieve these, and what barriers you might need to cross or deal with as you go.

Consider that there are many different ways to help you achieve your goals. You might like to join a yoga or tai chi class, start walking with a friend, or just take some quiet space in each day to 'drop anchor' and calm your mind.

Finally, pick a date to get started, tell your close friends or partners about your plan so they can keep a check on you, and go for it!

Remember, setbacks are normal, and watch yourself for unhelpful 'all or nothing' thinking. Most things that are worthwhile are effort, but if you never start, you most certainly will not get there.

continued over page …

Goal: ______________________________

Short Term Milestones	*Medium Term Milestones*
______________	______________
______________	______________
______________	______________
When will I get there?	*When will I get there?*
______________	______________
______________	______________
______________	______________
How do I get there?	*How do I get there?*
______________	______________
______________	______________
______________	______________
Who do I need?	*Who do I need?*
______________	______________
______________	______________
What do I need?	*What do I need?*
______________	______________
______________	______________
Barriers	*Barriers*
______________	______________
______________	______________

Tiger Activity Handout 5

FACING THE TIGER

Treatment Decision Making

(See *Facing the Tiger* Chapter 5, page 58.)

Make a list of the treatments your doctor has suggested would be suitable for you. Beside each option list the possible positives (the pros) and the possible negatives (the cons).

Treatment 1: ____________________________

Pros	*Cons*

Treatment 2: ____________________________

Pros	*Cons*

Treatment3: ______________________________

Pros	*Cons*
______________________	______________________
______________________	______________________
______________________	______________________
______________________	______________________
______________________	______________________

Looking at the pros and cons for each, does it look like one option has more pros and fewer cons than the others?

Now put a circle around the pros that matter to you most and the cons that worry you the most. What option looks like it will get you what you value most?

Take this list to your doctor and talk it over with him to make sure you have the facts right. Talk the list over with your partner or someone close to you that you trust. This will help you clarify further what option seems to be closest to your values and will keep your support network in the loop.

Tiger Activity Handout 6

Problem Solving

(See *Facing the Tiger* Chapter 9, page 119.)

Make a list of the main problems that are worrying you right now. Do this separately on your own and then share these with your partner. Do you have some problems that you both are concerned about and could work on together? Are there things worrying your partner that you were unaware of?

Problem	***Priority***
	☐
	☐
	☐
	☐
	☐

Pick off your top three priorities and ask yourself if you understand clearly how this problem has arisen. If you need more information about the problem, make a decision to find out more. Once you feel you are well informed, generate a list of possible actions you could take to help with each priority and consider which actions you feel comfortable doing and most confident about. Think about who can help you with this and what extra support you might need, and what milestones you want to reach and when.

Priority: ____________________________________

How did this problem arise?

____

____

____

Possible actions

____

____

____

____

Support

____

____

____

Milestones

____

____

____

____

Now you have a plan, you can move into action. Remember however that if all does not go the way you planned or hoped, it is okay to reconsider and revise the plan.

Tiger Activity Handout 7

Automatic Thinking

(See *Facing the Tiger* Chapter 7, page 82.)

Most of the time we think in an automatic way, without effort, and in patterns we have learned and practised all our lives. How many times have you reflected that someone you know (or maybe even you) always thinks the worst, or the best, or jumps to conclusions? It matters because we do tend to respond as if our thoughts are absolutely true, and if our mind perceives a tiger out there, our bodies will react as if there really is one and will set off the physical stress response accordingly. You can test this out for yourself in the following simple thinking exercise.

First, think about something that happened in the past that was really upsetting. Remind yourself where this was, who was there and think about what happened and what was said. Think and remember what happened.

How do you feel right now after thinking about this?

____

____

____

____

Now think about something that you would really like to happen, something you have dreamed about. Who would be there with you, and where would you be?

What feelings do these thoughts and images bring up in you at this moment?

____

____

____

____

For both of these exercises, the reality of who and where you are right now didn't change, but how you feel probably did. The only thing that did change was what you were thinking about. How we think and what we think about affects how we feel.

Tiger Activity Handout 8

Identifying Patterns of Thinking

(See *Facing the Tiger* Chapter 7, page 86.)

For the next week, keep notes in your journal of the times when you find yourself feeling more upset or stressed. Jot down the day and time, where you are and who you are with, what is going on and most importantly, what you are thinking and feeling. Use the layout below.

- Day & Time:
- Where was I?
- Who was I with?
- What was happening?
- What was I thinking and feeling?

After a week of keeping these notes, take some time to look them over and see if you can identify a pattern. Do you have a typical way of thinking that you can identify? Are there any of the negative common thinking patterns mentioned in the book (pages 83–84). Are your thoughts realistic or based on accurate or true and known information? Are these thoughts helping or hindering you? Is there a way you could think about what is happening that would serve you better?

Talk this over if you can with your partner or a close and trusted friend. Ask them to support you in coming up with a more helpful view of what is going on. If you don't feel you can talk about these thoughts with someone else, or just prefer not to, become your own best friend. Write down a different way to look at the problem or challenge you are facing that expresses kindness and care to yourself.

Now, find some time in the next week to sit in the garden or go for a short walk. As you do this, notice what is around you. Focus your attention on the finer details of the trees or plants, how the wind plays with your surroundings, and how the sunlight falls and changes the colours around you. Are there small animals you notice, ants or lizards? What noises can you hear? Is there traffic in the distance, can you hear laughter in the background and the sounds of your own breathing? Now notice how you feel. Practice using this grounding technique next time that you notice getting carried away with negative thoughts.

Tiger Activity Handout 9

Getting Unstuck

(See *Facing the Tiger* Chapter 10, page 130.)

In life, we all have our stories. About how we grew up, the good and bad things that have happened to us, the people who helped and the people who hindered, the things we are proud of and what we might regret. Woven together, this becomes our story or *narrative* about who we are, how our life generally plays out, what we hope for, what we strive for, what we expect, and what we need to live.

Sometimes though, life throws us a curveball. We find that the narrative we have been working with doesn't seem to help us. We can't seem to move forward or get over the speed bump. In other words, we get stuck. If you are feeling 'stuck', this might mean that you need a different approach to how you are looking at your cancer diagnosis and your future and how you sit in the world. This counts for men with prostate cancer and their partners equally.

Perhaps you are feeling anxious a lot of the time and are finding it hard to relax and feel easy in your skin. You might be living with a sense of grief and loss that is weighing you down — or worrying a lot of the time about the future and what it could hold. Maybe you are angry or annoyed more than you would like or feel that your relationships are not working as well as they might. These two things might be linked. You might also be feeling a need for more direction in your life or a shift to a different purpose.

But first, you need to decide if you are really up for change and what that might mean, and what yearnings or past grievances you might need to let go of. This starts with awareness and reflection about your narrative for how you got to this point in life and what that narrative means to you. Doing the same thing repeatedly will generally lead to the same outcome. Is your current approach serving you well? Are you up for considering change? If yes, the first step is awareness.

Awareness

Set aside some time when you won't be interrupted. Find a comfortable place to sit where your body is well supported and relaxed. Start by building awareness of your breath. Gently place your hands on your belly. If you feel relaxed to do so, close your eyes. Breathe slowly to a count of four for each in-breath and each out-breath. Notice the breath coming into your body through your nose, the temperature of the air as you draw this into your body. Notice how your belly expands as you breathe in and relaxes back as you breathe out. Maintain this focus on your breath and direct your attention to this sensation.

Now start to notice other parts of your body and how they feel. The soles of your feet and what they are placed upon, the pressure you feel there. Notice your posture and whether it is tight or loose. Gently move your shoulders and check for tension in your neck. Notice how your facial muscles are feeling, is your brow relaxed? Is your jaw tight or loose?

As you are doing this, your mind might wander to the worries of the day or the jobs and tasks you have to do and that are on your mind. Notice these thoughts and the feelings that come with them, and how these thoughts affect your body tension. These thoughts and feelings are not in and of themselves good or bad; they just are what they are. Notice them, be aware of them, and now gently direct your attention back to your breath.

Now listen to the sounds you can hear around you. This might be traffic noises, or birds, wind in the trees, household noises. This is where you are right now, in the present.

So now, in the present moment, turn to your heart and your head. What changes are you looking for in how you sit in the present? What would this mean for you? What words describe how this would look and feel?

When you are ready, focus again on counting in for four and out for four on each breath, and then open your eyes and jot down the feelings and thoughts you became aware of and the changes that you are looking for in your present moment or situation. Use the prompts below.

Exercise: Where I am right now

Feelings

Feelings I often experience that are difficult or uncomfortable to sit with.

____

____

____

____

How do I express these feelings to myself and to those close to me?

____

____

____

____

____

Thoughts

Thoughts that tend to come with these difficult or uncomfortable feelings.

____

____

____

____

What do I think might be the source of these thoughts? Do I treat these thoughts as if they are absolute truths? As facts that are certain and can't be changed?

Is there a way I can talk or speak about these thoughts and see them as just thoughts? Look at them from a distance as if they were a story I had been told a long time ago?

Exercise: Who am I?

If I were able to look at myself as if I were a bystander to my life as it is right now, what would I see?

What advice would I give to myself if I were my own best and trusted friend? Speaking to myself as a compassionate adviser, what would I say?

____

____

____

____

____

Making Choices

How we live is up to all of us. Life will have delivered highs and lows, successes and losses. Rarely is this all good or all bad. It is the tapestry, it is our story or narrative, and we can become fused or glued to the past and our expectations of the future as if it is the only possible reality. We can get stuck in our past thoughts, feelings and behaviours and our expectations that this is all there is or can be.

But how you experience the world and those around you *can* change into the future. Dwelling on the past is not likely to lead to change. Living in the present can lessen the burden of the past, and deciding to make changes for the future brings with it possibilities. No one is perfect, none of us. So, accepting that and letting go of 'what ifs' and 'I should have' or 'might have' can be very freeing. It is about opening up to possibility, dropping self-blame, suspending judgement of ourselves and those around us, and responding to what we see and experience in new ways.

Small changes can make important differences in how closely we connect with people who are important to us, and in how we walk in the future with ourselves in a spirit of self-compassion — being the self that we want to be and connecting with others the way we want to.

Exercise: Where I want to be

What are the key areas of my life and how I am in the present that I would like to change? What do I hope for? What matters to me most now?

____

____

____

____

____

What thoughts or feelings are holding me back that would I need to step aside from to give myself a chance for change?

____

____

____

____

____

Trying out Change

Change is hard. Most of us tend to avoid it. A good place to start is to think of some small steps or actions towards how you want your life to be and set yourself up with these as experiments you can try. For example, if you have relationships that you would like to deepen and appreciate more, what might be an action you could take towards this? Perhaps there are activities you have always felt would be fun and rewarding but that you have avoided because of embarrassment or fear or never managing to find the time. Maybe you haven't felt you had earned the chance for change or something new or better. Make a list of things you have always wanted to try that align with how you would like most to be or what matters most in your present life. Select five new activities or behaviours to start with. Think of this as an experiment for acting and feeling differently. Lean in. Try saying 'yes'.

Exercise: Where I want to be

List five new activities or behaviours you would like to try, for example, meeting up with a good friend you haven't seen for some time, listening again to the music you most loved in your younger years, enjoying a good movie. Look for a short course on a topic you have always wanted to know more about. It's your list — what would expand your life?

1. ________________________________

2. ________________________________

3. ________________________________

4. ________________________________

5. ________________________________

Now schedule each of these activities to try out over the next six weeks. Commit yourself 100%. No self-evaluation or criticism is allowed. This is an experiment for you in widening out your range and view of what is possible in your life.

Worksheet

FACING THE TIGER

Masculinity in Health Inventory[1]

The following is a series of statements men have told us are important for them in thinking about their health and well-being. There are no right or wrong answers to these questions. The purpose here is to reflect on values that might be important to you and might be influencing how you are feeling right now.

Thinking about you personally, please indicate how true each statement is for you on a scale of 1 "not at all true", 3 "somewhat true" to 5 "very true". There are no right or wrong answers. Please give the responses that most accurately describe your personal thoughts and feelings.

		Not at all true	A little true	Somewhat true	Mostly true	Very true
1.	Being physically strong is important to me	1	2	3	4	5
2.	I feel and think young	1	2	3	4	5
3.	I get frustrated when things progress slowly	1	2	3	4	5
4.	I am a carefree person	1	2	3	4	5
5.	Being physically able to have sex is important to me	1	2	3	4	5
6.	I always look for the good in situations	1	2	3	4	5
7.	I keep my feelings to myself	1	2	3	4	5
8.	Being able to have an erection is important to me	1	2	3	4	5
9.	I like to take action in the face of problems	1	2	3	4	5
10.	I like to win	1	2	3	4	5
11.	I like to know I am looking after my partner or family	1	2	3	4	5
12.	Having a good level of fitness is important to me	1	2	3	4	5
13.	I am a fighter	1	2	3	4	5
14.	If I want to achieve something I can	1	2	3	4	5
15.	I like to know I am capable of having sex	1	2	3	4	5

continued over page ...

[1]Chambers, S. K., Hyde, M. K., Oliffe, J. L., Zajdlewicz, L., Lowe, A., Wootten, A. C., & Dunn, J. (2015). Measuring masculinity in the context of chronic disease. Psychology of Men and Masculinity.

		Not at all true	A little true	Somewhat true	Mostly true	Very true
16.	I am a positive person	1	2	3	4	5
17.	I tend not to talk about my worries	1	2	3	4	5
18.	I like to know I can father a child if I want to	1	2	3	4	5
19.	I like to be in control	1	2	3	4	5
20.	I need to provide financial security for my partner or family	1	2	3	4	5
21.	Being an active person is important to me	1	2	3	4	5
22.	I overdo things at times	1	2	3	4	5
23.	I have a forward thinking mind set	1	2	3	4	5
24.	I like to take risks	1	2	3	4	5
25.	Being able to have sex is like being able to run	1	2	3	4	5
26.	Being able to provide for my partner or family is important to me	1	2	3	4	5
27.	I am optimistic about the future	1	2	3	4	5
28.	I am a competitive person	1	2	3	4	5
29.	My approach is to get on with things	1	2	3	4	5
30.	It is up to me to protect my partner or family	1	2	3	4	5

Reflection Points

Now, in looking over your answers, consider if some values you hold strongly can help you with your current concerns. For example, can you use a 'can-do' self-reliant approach to seek help for current problems and make and follow an action plan? If you tend to keep worries close to yourself, can you identify someone you can share your concerns with to take some pressure off yourself? If you tend to overdo things or get frustrated with slow progress, is this serving you well right now, and is there an alternative way to look at things in the present? Values about fitness and being active can be used as a motivator towards accessing exercise medicine for both strength and mental wellbeing. If partner and family relationships are important, this can be a priority for the future.

Tiger Activity Handout 10

Getting Sex Back on Track

(See *Facing the Tiger* Chapter 5, page 72.)

Set aside time to talk about how you are each feeling about your sexual lives and how you would like things to be in the best of worlds. This is best not done in the bedroom, where you might each feel a little tense. Try talking about this over a cup of coffee or a relaxing drink after dinner. You need privacy and to pick a time when you won't be interrupted. The goal here is to agree on what steps you would like to take as a couple to get sex back on track. Once you agree, you can start to make a plan about what external medical help you would like, get informed about the options, and try out options that suit you both. Think of your options as a menu (perhaps French!) to choose from. Be prepared to try different approaches until you find one that you are both happy with.

When you are trying to get back to a normal sex life, it helps to start by making time to give each other physical, sensual pleasure without having actual sex. For this activity sexual touch is banned! Set aside at least one hour for private physical touch time. You need a private place like your bedroom, there needs to be no interruptions, and you both need to agree that the next hour (or two) is for giving and receiving pleasure through physical touch. Candles, soft mood lighting and relaxing music is a good start as well as a state of undress to the extent you are comfortable. Now take turns touching and massaging your partner in non-sexual places, fifteen to twenty minute turns each. Notice how good it feels to touch and be touched, and to give and receive pleasure. Talk to each other (compliments are good) and have fun with this. This exercise is about being close and feeling good about yourself and each other.

When you are comfortable with touching in places that are less 'sexual', try different ways of giving and receiving sensual pleasure short of having actual sexual intercourse. This can include touching each other on sensitive and sexual parts of the body and giving pleasure through physical stimulation using hands or your mouth. Be playful. Instead of worrying about reaching an orgasm, just focus on learning new ways to give each other pleasure. Ask each other what feels good and work on learning what kinds of touch your partner prefers. For this exercise, sexual intercourse is not the goal. The goal is finding ways to give sexual or sensual pleasure to each other that do not rely on having an erection or achieving penetration. It is about intimacy and trust.

Prostate Cancer Distress Screen

Use the QR code link below to download a free PDF copy of the Prostate Cancer Distress Screen from the Prostate Cancer Foundation of Australia website.

https://pcfa.org.au/media/790557/pcfa-distress-screening-tool-september-2019.pdf

Appendix 4

Prostate Cancer Survivorship Care Plan

You are free to photocopy the Prostate Cancer Survivorship Care Plan on the following pages (it will reproduce best at a magnification of 125%) or use the QR code link below to download a PDF form copy from the publisher. This form is able to be filled in and printed out using a range of freely available PDF reader apps such as Adobe Acrobat Reader (or Apple Preview if you are running Mac OS). An email address is required to immediately begin the download.

https://sowl.co/QMQXc

My Personal Plan

PROSTATE CANCER SURVIVORSHIP ESSENTIALS

A Survivorship Plan is a summary of information about your diagnosis, treatment and ongoing care. You can take this with you to any future health care appointments so that any care providers involved in your current and future care have a clear picture of your diagnosis and treatment. Ask a member of your Prostate Cancer healthcare team to assist you in completing your Survivorship Plan and ensure you keep this up to date.

My Details

Name

Care Plan Start Date

Treating Specialist

Treating Hospital/Centre

Prostate Cancer Specialist Nurse

General Practitioner

My Diagnosis

Date of Diagnosis

My Treatment Plan

Complete any areas that apply to you.

Surgery

Surgery date:

Treating Hospital /Centre:

Procedure:

Complications:

Comments:

Radiation Therapy

Start date:

Treating Hospital:

Site (e.g. prostate, hip):

Number of Treatments:

Side Effects:

Comments:

Hormone Therapy

Start date:

Treating Hospital /Centre:

Therapy Type:

Treatment Term:

Side Effects:

Comments:

Brachytherapy

Start date:

Treating Hospital:

LDR or HDR:

Side Effects:

Comments:

Chemotherapy / Targeted Therapy

Start date:

Treating Hospital /Centre:

Therapy Type:

Number of Treatments:

Side Effects:

Comments:

Active Surveillance

Start date:

Treating Hospital /Centre:

Next PSA test:

Next scan:

Next biopsy:

Comments:

Medications

If not stated already please list any medications you are currently taking that are related to Prostate Cancer treatment or symptoms:

Follow Up Appointments

Please list any follow up appointments you have scheduled:

Date	Specialist	Tests required	Comments

Additional Information

Please note any additional information that is relevant to your diagnosis or treatment e.g., PSA levels, Active Surveillance Plan, etc.

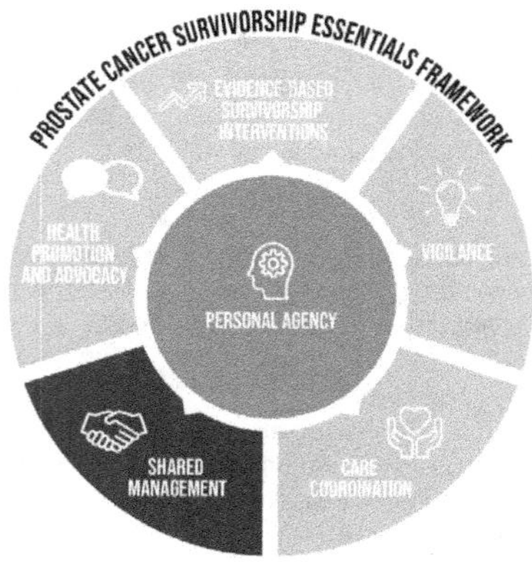

My Wellbeing Plan

For most men having prostate cancer leads to some changes in wellbeing. The type of changes and how long they persist will depend on the types of treatments you receive and your overall health. There are evidence-based interventions that you can use to help self-manage or minimise these effects and your doctor or nurse can advise you about this. This plan includes a list of some possible effects and who can help. Any person who has had a cancer diagnosis is considered to be a survivor. Survivorship care means having a plan to look after your wellbeing now and for any changes that might happen in the future. It's all about you!

There are six areas to consider:

1. Personal agency

Personal agency means taking control about what help you need, and seeking support to manage your own health where you can. This does not mean going it alone, it means finding out who is there to help, what you can do yourself and what others can offer, and being an active part of the team.

What can I do?

✓ *Set survivorship goals that most matter to you. In thinking of the months and years ahead, what are the health and wellbeing goals that you would like to work towards. These might be goals around physical activity or mental wellbeing, you may also have goals around urinary control or other physical symptoms. Strengthening your intimate relationship or perhaps looking to develop one might be on your list. Once you have your goals clear then identify the information and other support you might need to achieve these goals. Set targets that are achievable and put an action plan in place with a timeline. Be prepared to be flexible and problem solve as you go along. This approach will help you to feel more in control of your care.*

2. Shared management

Shared management means being an equal partner in your health care, sharing decision making with your health care team and sharing how you will tackle challenges as they arise. This includes informed decision making around testing and treatment, understanding and managing the physical and psychological effects of treatment and of the disease.

What can I do?

✓ *Let your health care team know how involved you want to be in decisions about your care, and who else you want to be involved, such as your partner or other family or friends. Question lists can help guide the conversation with your doctor, nurse or other health professional and ensure you ask about the things that matter most to you. Plan in advance what questions you need answered, perhaps with the support of a partner or a close friend.*

✓ *Make sure your General Practitioner is connected into your care so that they are well prepared to support you.*

3. Vigilance

Your health care provider will manage surveillance from diagnosis and through life, and this includes physical issues such as the control of the cancer and management of physical side effects but also other illnesses that can occur as we age. This also includes checking on your emotional and social wellbeing.

What can I do?

✓ *Ask your doctor about your check-up schedule going forward and keep a record of this using this care plan.*
✓ *Communicate your concerns and how you are going physically and emotionally to your health care team.*
✓ *Your psychological wellbeing is just as important as your physical health. Use the scale and problem list below to gauge your level of stress.*

A quick way to gauge your level of stress is to is to ask yourself how distressed have you felt over the past week on a scale of 0 (no distress), to 10 (extreme distress)? If you are 4 or over on this scale then your doctor or nurse needs to know so they can work with you on what support you might need. If you are 4 or over on this scale then your doctor or nurse needs to know so they can work with you on what support you might need.

Click or check the number to score how distressed you have felt in the last week:

No distress

0
1
2
3
4
5
6
7
8
9
10

Extreme distress

Check the items on the list below to get a sense of what might be most strongly influencing how you are feeling:

Practical problems

Work

Financial/insurance

Family problems

Partner

Emotional problems

Depression

Uncertainty about the future

Nervousness

Sadness

Worry

Loss of interest in usual activities

Treatment problems

Understanding treatments

Making a decision

Information about my illness

Physical problems

Pain

Fatigue

Sexual

Urinary

Bowel

Hot flushes

Weight gain

Weight loss

Loss of muscle mass

Memory/concentration

Sleep

Other problems (please list)

Talk to your doctor or nurse about the problem that is concerning you the most to find out what services are available to you and how you can access them.

4. Evidence-based survivorship interventions

Your time and energy are valuable. Being evidence-based is about directing your time, energy and resources to strategies that have strong evidence to support their effectiveness. There is excellent evidence for the benefits of exercise medicine. For overall wellness good nutritional habits are important. Psychological support helps manage mood changes and the stress and anxiety associated with cancer. Sexual health support tailored to individual men in different age groups and with different sexual orientations and relationships is also an area where good evidence exists about what works.

What can I do?

- ✓ *Check with your doctor or nurse or organisations such as the Prostate Cancer Foundation of Australia about what services are available for you.*
- ✓ *Talk to other men who have had prostate cancer to see what they have found helpful and accessible, support groups can help here.*
- ✓ *Ask your General Practitioner to help with Medicare support for service through a Chronic Disease Management Plan for allied health services, or the Better Access to Mental Health for psychology.*

5. Care coordination

Care Coordination is about your health care team working together to get you the best care possible in a 'right place at the right time' approach.

What can I do?

- ✓ *Ask your doctor or nurse who is the lead person coordinating your care and how you can contact them if you need to. Also ask who is keeping your General Practitioner in the loop. If you move to a different treatment approach you might need to ask this again.*

6. Health promotion and advocacy

Having accurate and up to date information about prostate cancer is important for you, your family and your community.

What can I do?

- ✓ *Be informed and active in seeking information about your cancer and your health care from credible and reliable sources.*
- ✓ *Share what you know about prostate cancer with people who matter to you, your partner and family and close networks.*
- ✓ *Reach out to local support prostate cancer support groups in your area.*

Your referrals

The following is a list of services that may assist you in your Prostate Cancer recovery journey. Please tick any services that you have engaged with. If you are interested in any of these services, ask your treating team or GP for a referral.

	Referred	**On-going treatment**	**No longer required**
Psychology			
Social work			
Sexual counselling			
Psychiatry			
Pain or palliative care			
Continence support			
Genetic counselling			
Dietician			
Physiotherapy			
Occupational therapy			
Fertility			
Prostate nurse			
Smoking cessation			
Other			

Supplementary health services

Services such as allied health professionals can assist with your recovery from Prostate Cancer symptoms and treatment, as well as benefiting your overall health and wellbeing. In order to access these services, speak to your GP or your treating team at the hospital. Your doctors can provide you with a referral to public or private services that may benefit you. Services include:

- **Exercise Physiology** provides tailored clinical exercise interventions to manage symptoms associated with prostate cancer treatment and improve functional performance. Interventions also include health and physical activity information, and support for lifestyle modifications and behavioural change. You can find out more about exercise physiology at: https://exerciseright.com.au/what-is-an-accredited-exercise-physiologist/

- **Dietetics** provides personalised nutrition advice and support including eating plans, advice on supplements and nutritional counselling. You can find out more about dietetics at: https://dietitiansaustralia.org.au/what-dietitans-do/

- **Psychology** services provide support and treatment for anxiety, depression and distress, and other psychological concerns related to cancer. You can find out more about psychology at: https://www.psychology.org.au/for-the-public/about-psychology

- **Physiotherapy** helps strengthen the body, improve mobility and manage pain after prostate cancer treatment using movement and exercise, manual therapy, education and advice. You can find out more about physiotherapy at: https://choose.physio/what-is-physio

- **Occupational therapy** provides support if you are having difficulty with everyday tasks and helps you maintain, regain or improve your independence. You can find out more about occupational therapy at: https://otaus.com.au/about/about-ot

- **Social work** offers counselling services, therapeutic interventions, and information and resources for patients, families and carers to support decision making and access services and support. You can find out more about social work at: https://www.aasw.asn.au/information-for-the-community/information-for-the-community

Other Helpful Services

- **Prostate Cancer Foundation of Australia (PCFA)** is the peak national body for prostate cancer in Australia and supports men and their families affected by prostate cancer through evidence-based information and resources, support groups and Prostate Cancer Specialist Nurses: https://www.prostate.org.au/

- **Prostate Cancer Specialist Telenursing Service**: This service, provided by the Prostate Cancer Foundation of Australia (PCFA), connects you to a Prostate Cancer Specialist Nurse who can help you with evidence-based information, practical and emotional support, and can link you with local support networks: https://www.prostate.org.au/support/prostate-cancer-specialist-telenursing-service/

  To access this service you can:
  - ✓ Phone: 1800 22 00 99
  - ✓ Email: telenurse@pcfa.org.au
  - ✓ Submit an online form: https://www.prostate.org.au/telenursing-request-form/

  If you have a *hearing or speech impairment*, call the National Relay Service on 1800 555 677 and ask to be transferred to PCFA's Telenursing Service at 1800 22 00 99. If *English is not your main language* and you need an interpreter, call TIS National on 131 450 and ask to be transferred to PCFA's Telenursing Service at 1800 22 00 99.

Dunn J, Green A, Ralph N, Newton R, Kneebone A, Frydenberg M, Chambers SK. Prostate Cancer Survivorship Essentials Framework: Guidelines for Practitioners. BJUI. 2020; https://doi.org/10.1111/bju.15159.

Chambers SK. Facing the Tiger: A Survivorship Guide for Men with Prostate Cancer and their Partners. Brisbane, Australia: Australian Academic Press; 2020.

Appendix 5

Patient Screening Tools

You are free to photocopy the resources following in this Appendix:

- Patient Health Questionnaire (PHQ-9)
- Generalised Anxiety Disorder Assessment (GAD-7)

or use the QR code link below to access the Pfizer Patient Health Questionnaire website where you can download both screening instruments as well as scoring information.

https://www.phqscreeners.com/

Appendix 5.1 Patient Health Questionnaire (PHQ-9)*

Appendix 5.2 Generalised Anxiety Disorder Assessment (GAD-7)**

* Kroenke K, Spitzer RL, Williams JB. The PHQ-9: validity of a brief depression severity measure. Journal of General Internal Medicine. 2001;16(9):606-13.

** Spitzer RL, Kroenke K, Williams JB, Löwe B. A brief measure for assessing generalized anxiety disorder: the GAD-7. Archives of Internal Medicine. 2006;166(10):1092-7.

PATIENT HEALTH QUESTIONNAIRE-9 (PHQ-9)

Over the previous 2 weeks, how often have you been bothered by any of the following problems? *(Use "✔" to indicate your answer)*	**Not at all**	**Several days**	**More than half of the two week period**	**Nearly every day**
1. Little pleasure or little interest in doing things	0	1	2	3
2. Feeling down, depressed, or hopeless	0	1	2	3
3. Trouble falling or staying asleep, or sleeping too much	0	1	2	3
4. Having little energy or feeling tired	0	1	2	3
5. Poor appetite or overeating	0	1	2	3
6. Feeling negative about yourself or that you are a failure or have let your self or your family down	0	1	2	3
7. Trouble concentrating on things, such as reading the newspaper or watching television	0	1	2	3
8. Moving or talking so slowly that other people could have noticed? Or the opposite — being so fidgety or restless that you have been moving around a lot more than usual	0	1	2	3
9. Thoughts that you would be better off dead or of hurting yourself in some way	0	1	2	3

FOR OFFICE CODING __*0*__ + ______ + ______ + ______

=Total Score: ______

If you ticked off any of the problems above, how difficult has it been for you to do your work, take care of things at home or get along with other people because of these problems?

Not difficult at all	**Somewhat difficult**	**Very difficult**	**Extremely difficult**
☐	☐	☐	☐

Developed by Drs. Robert L. Spitzer, Janet B.W. Williams, Kurt Kroenke and colleagues, with an educational grant from Pfizer Inc. No permission required to reproduce, translate, display or distribute.

GAD-7

Over the <u>last two weeks</u>, how often have you been bothered by the following problems? *(Use ☐✔☐ to indicate your answer)*	Not at all	Several days	More than half the days	Nearly every day
1. Feeling nervous, anxious or on edge	0	1	2	3
2. Not being able to stop or control worrying	0	1	2	3
3. Worrying too much about different things	0	1	2	3
4. Having trouble relaxing	0	1	2	3
5. Being so restless that it is hard to sit still	0	1	2	3
6. Becoming easily annoyed or irritable	0	1	2	3
7. Feeling afraid as if something awful might happen	0	1	2	3

(*For office coding: Total Score T_____ = ___ + ___ + ___*)

Developed by Drs. Robert L. Spitzer, Janet B.W. Williams, Kurt Kroenke and colleagues, with an educational grant from Pfizer, Inc. No permission required to reproduce, translate, display or distribute.

Facing the Tiger

Each man with whom you are conducting an intervention built from this Guide will require a copy of the self-help book *Facing the Tiger: A Survivorship Guide for Men with Prostate Cancer and their Partners.* The book is available from the publisher's webstore (www.aapbooks.com) as well as most major online bookstores and on order from local bookstores.

For your reference and private use when preparing intervention sessions, a complete copy of *Facing the Tiger* is reproduced on the following pages.

FACING
THE TIGER

Professor Suzanne Chambers AO
PHD MAPS

AUSTRALIANACADEMIC**PRESS**

First published 2020 by:
Australian Academic Press Group Pty. Ltd.
Samford Valley, Australia
www.australianacademicpress.com.au

Copyright © 2020 Suzanne Chambers

Reprinted 2021

The author has donated all royalties due from the sale of this book to the Prostate Cancer Foundation of Australia. www.prostate.org.au

Copying for educational purposes
The *Australian Copyright Act 1968* (Cwlth) allows a maximum of one chapter or 10% of this book, whichever is the greater, to be reproduced and/or communicated by any educational institution for its educational purposes provided that the educational institution (or the body that administers it) has given a remuneration notice to Copyright Agency Limited (CAL) under the Act.

For details of the CAL licence for educational institutions contact:
Copyright Agency Limited, 19/157 Liverpool Street, Sydney, NSW 2000.
E-mail info@copyright.com.au

Production and communication for other purposes
Except as permitted under the Act, for example a fair dealing for the purposes of study, research, criticism or review, no part of this book may be reproduced, stored in a retrieval system, or transmitted in any form or by any means electronic, mechanical, photocopying, recording or otherwise without prior written permission of the copyright holder.

NATIONAL LIBRARY OF AUSTRALIA

A catalogue record for this book is available from the National Library of Australia

Facing the Tiger: A Survivorship Guide for Men with Prostate Cancer and their Partners
ISBN 9781925644425 (paperback)
ISBN 9781925644432 (ebook)

DISCLAIMER: Every effort has been made in preparing this work to provide information based on accepted evidence, standards and practice at the time of publication. By referring to this book, any and all readers release the author and publisher of any claims of direct or consequential damages resulting from relying on the content contained herein.

Publisher & Editor: Stephen May

Cover design: Luke Harris, Working Type Studio

Typesetting: Australian Academic Press

Printing: Lightning Source

To order bulk copies of this book please email
orders@australianacademicpress.com.au

Praise for *Facing the Tiger*

'Professor Suzanne Chambers is a highly regarded, experienced and practical researcher and practitioner in the management of psychological issues that emerge when a man is diagnosed with cancer of the prostate. The diagnosis not only affects him but invariably impacts his partner, family and friends.

This book clearly identifies key issues and provides reassurance and solutions in a compact, readable style that immediately puts the reader at ease and empowers them to "face the tiger".

Each chapter includes specific activities to address the issues discussed and is rounded off with personal stories not only from survivors of prostate cancer but their partners and families as well. Two new chapters in this edition "Getting Unstuck" and "Survivorship" are valuable additions as they speak to the longer term. We cannot forget that at the time of publication over 200,000 men are living with prostate cancer in Australia. Over 95% of men diagnosed with prostate cancer will be alive five years after diagnosis and treatment.

The appendix contains well selected, trusted, quality resources for men, their partners and families and friends to start their own research to compliment the book.

Nearly 20,000 men a year are diagnosed with and 3500 men die from prostate cancer in Australia each year. The diagnosis and management of prostate cancer constitutes a significant proportion of modern Urological practice. This book will be an invaluable resource for Urologists and all clinicians involved in the diagnosis and management of prostate cancer, not only in Australia and New Zealand but around the world.'

— **Peter Heathcote**, *Former President Urological Society of Australia and New Zealand, Adjunct Professor Australian Prostate Cancer Research Centre Queensland, Queensland University of Technology, Adjunct Clinical Professor Monash University Public Health and Preventive Medicine, Senior Urologist Princess Alexandra Hospital, Brisbane, Australia*

'I thoroughly endorse this book as being essential reading for any man who has been diagnosed with prostate cancer, his partner, and his medical personnel. The psychosocial effects from the management of this disease has long represented one of the seriously unmet needs.

Suzanne Chambers, as a psychologist with a doctorate in the psychosocial management of men diagnosed with prostate cancer, and a confidante who helped me set up the Brisbane prostate cancer support group in Queensland, is now a recognised international authority on this subject. This is a book I would have loved to have access to when I was diagnosed, in 1996.'

— **Peter Dornan AM**, *Physiotherapist, writer, sculptor, 2020 Senior Australian of the Year for Queensland, 'Men's Health Advocate'.*

'Being diagnosed with prostate cancer begins a journey no man — or his partner — wishes to take. But if fate finds you on it, Professor Suzanne Chambers' book will guide you. In clear and approachable prose and with real-world stories, *Facing the Tiger* not only points out the twists and turns, it also gives you practical advice on how to become a stronger, more confident man, a more supportive and effective partner. I highly recommend it.'

— **Mark Lazenby, PhD,** *Fellow of the American Psychosocial Oncology Society and of the American Academy of Nursing; Professor of Nursing and Philosophy, University of Connecticut, USA.*

'There is probably no optimum way to face a tiger just as there is more than one way to face a diagnosis of prostate cancer. In this book Suzanne Chambers brings her expertise as a psychologist who has helped people deal with cancer together with the experience of men, their partners and families who have had to deal with a prostate cancer diagnosis. In doing so I believe that Suzanne has provided a resource in which many men and their families will find comfort and reassurance that others have managed to deal with the challenges presented by a diagnosis of prostate cancer.

Given the choices that are faced regarding treatment I think the chapter on decision making is particularly relevant whilst this and the advice on exercise and general wellbeing echo a lot of what we are seeking to do at Prostate Scotland. This book may not provide all of the answers or help that every man and their families need, but I am sure it will help many.'

— **Prof. Alan McNeill,** *Consultant Urological Surgeon (Western General Hospital Edinburgh), Hon. Professor in the School of Engineering and physical Sciences Heriot Watt University, Trustee of Prostate Scotland*

'*Facing The Tiger* raises psycho-social help to a new level for all prostate cancer patients. Inclusion and empathy form the spine of this helpful guidebook for emotional support. It is required reading for all men with prostate cancer.'

— **Darryl Mitteldorf, LCSW,** *Director, Malecare Cancer Support, New York, NY*

'Suzanne Chambers has been a long-time world leader in psychosocial prostate cancer — and the revised edition of Facing the Tiger is an exceptional offering that will significantly advance the knowledge of men (and their partners) who encounter prostate cancer. Offered are testimonials that share important experiences across the typical sequence of diagnosis, treatment decision making and recovery. Threaded through these patient and partner experiences are practical strategies for recognizing and dealing effectively with the challenges that inevitably come with prostate cancer. In addition to adjustments for sexual function there is a focus on avenues for achieving and sustaining overall mental and physical health. Informed by world leading research Facing the Tiger is a must have easy- to-read resource that will inform and empower all who are exposed to prostate cancer.'

— **John Oliffe, PhD,** *Professor and Canada Research Chair (Tier 1) in Men's Health Promotion, University of British Columbia*

'Prostate cancer and its treatments have potential complications and side effects on physical aspects of a man's quality of life such as continence and erectile function. The psychological impact of a diagnosis of prostate cancer is sometimes overlooked in the clinician-patient relationship when considering decisions on prostate cancer management. Further, despite great advances in techniques to prevent or treat complications of prostate cancer treatment, results don't always fulfil expectations, resulting in considerable distress and sometimes decisional regret. This wonderful book is written by one of the world leaders in prostate cancer psychology research. This self-help book mixes evidence-based research with practical techniques to cope with the psychological diagnosis of prostate cancer. It also eloquently outlines the potential physical impact of prostate cancer progression or treatment side effects and provides important practical advice on management strategies. The personal stories highlight the importance of the impact prostate cancer has on the lives of men and their partners. I strongly recommend *Facing the Tiger* for all men and partners faced with the diagnosis of prostate cancer. I wish you well on your life long journey with this disease, but remember you are not alone and there is always someone available to help, please reach out and ask.'

— **Associate Professor John Yaxley,** *Wesley Urology Clinic, University of Queensland Department of Medicine, Royal Brisbane & Women's Hospital, Brisbane Australia*

'If you don't know where you want to go, you probably won't get there" argues Professor Suzanne Chambers playfully in this compact guide to prostate cancer survivorship. And then she promptly delivers clear directions to guide men with prostate cancer and their family and friends around the many challenges they might face. And while the advice is solidly grounded in the best available evidence, you do not have to take her word for it. Suzanne brings with her many diverse voices of men living with prostate cancer and their loved ones, to share their (sometimes hilarious) stories. This is not a medical textbook about cancer, this is a book about people affected by cancer who have so much more to share than just their cancer diagnosis. The chapters are brief, written in the breezy conversationalist style but full of tips and suggestions as well as realistic appraisal of what is easy and what many not be so. And the suggestions have broad applicability; how to grapple with difficult decisions, clarify your priorities, connect, and belong are just as relevant to prostate cancer survivorship as they are to other cancers. As the book points out, they are "what people with cancer have been asking for and doing themselves". Now, with Suzanne's expert help, the journey is clear!'

— **Professor Bogda Koczwara AM,** *Medical Oncologist and Cancer Survivorship Researcher, Flinders University, Adelaide, Australia*

'*Facing the Tiger* addresses prostate cancer from the patient's perspective — in the context of many men having a range of options for which there is no perfect answer. This book provides critical information empowering men to make personal choices based on their individual perspectives and priorities enabling them to choose their best path moving forward. The combination of evidence-based guidance with diverse personal stories makes for easy reading, with practical tips to empower patients to rationally choose a treatment option. This is a highly recommended resource for men with prostate cancer and those close to them.'

— **David Nicol,** *Chief of Surgery, Consultant Urological Surgeon, The Royal Marsden NHS Foundation Trust, Professor of Surgical Oncology, Institute of Cancer Research, UK*

'Prostate Cancer Foundation of Australia have been involved with this wonderful publication since its inception. It has been distributed and read by thousands of men and their families effected by a diagnosis of prostate cancer. The new personal stories and additional chapters will serve to reinforce and update all who will benefit from this new edition.'

— **Stephen Callister,** *National Chairman, Prostate Cancer Foundation of Australia , Adjunct Associate Professor, University of Technology Sydney*

Foreword

I've faced off against death once or twice in my life.

Going back a few years, I had a close call fishing on Moreton Bay, in Queensland with my old teammate Andrew Symonds. It was the middle of summer, and we'd set out before sunrise, dreaming about the catch.

Before we'd even wet a line, the ocean reminded us not to take anything for granted, throwing us over and sinking the boat.

Counter to what a lot of people say, my life didn't flash before my eyes. I could only see what was immediately in front of me. We simply went into survival mode. It was sink or swim.

In rough conditions and a little nervous of sharks, we somehow made it about a kilometre to shore, exhausted and in shock.

Before too long an old bloke who lived nearby saw us sitting there, shattered, on the beach.

Without any fuss, he extended his hand, 'Come to my place you silly buggers, I'll put the kettle on'.

I've never felt more comforted in my life.

Twenty years later, and I still remember how one bloke's kindness helped us feel hope and comfort through our shock.

As the son of a prostate cancer survivor, and a father facing the same risk, I recommend this book to you.

It is a powerful reminder that the future is always uncertain, but you're not alone in the struggle.

Matt Hayden AM
Managing Director
The Hayden Way

Acknowledgments

The first edition of this book was published in 2013 and was written at the request of men I had worked with who had experienced prostate cancer and who wanted a guide focussed on the day-to-day worries and concerns that they and their partners experience; hence *Facing the Tiger*. Today in 2020, some things about prostate cancer have changed, and others have not. The number of men affected has greatly increased, there are more specialised treatment options available, and there is greater awareness of the psychological and physical challenges men face. And yet, survivorship care for men and their partners and families remains in many cases fragmented so that men still report unmet needs and gaps in supportive care.

In updating this book to respond to the changes that have occurred and the problems that persist, I thank my partner Jeff Dunn for encouraging me to undertake a revision, and to continue to strive to make a difference. Thank you also to my research and clinical colleagues for further specialist advice, especially Rob Newton, Daniel Galvao and Samantha Clutton. To communications expert Anne Savage, my appreciation is always for your forthright comment and ongoing support. But mostly to the men who contributed new stories and updates to this book and who trusted my intent, my deep gratitude.

As before, the aim of this book is to provide a map to help you navigate your way through your cancer experience, and to develop an active approach to survivorship that works for you. The motto of remembering that everyone is different still stands true. Diversity can prompt new ways of looking at challenges that lead to new insights.

www.suzannechambers.com.au

Contents

Chapter 1

Facing the Tiger

Being told you have prostate cancer is, for most men and those close to them, an experience they will never forget. At that moment, the world seems changed. The things that you may have taken for granted are now at threat. While health care professionals and others around you may honestly express their concern and sympathy, this can be a singularly lonely and distressing time.

Once you experience a diagnosis of prostate cancer, you become a cancer survivor. You are not alone. Prostate cancer is now the most prevalent male cancer in the world, excluding non-melanoma skin cancer. In fact, if you take into account all cancers for both men and women, it is the third most prevalent cancer. The most recent estimates are that globally, based on five-year prevalence alone, more than 3,724,000 men are living with a diagnosis of prostate cancer. In the United States this includes over 737,000 men and similar numbers in Asia; in the United Kingdom over 206,000 men; and in Australia over 65,000 men. In Australia, there are now over 220,000 men who are living with a diagnosis of prostate cancer. This book aims to provide a map to help you see a way through this difficulty and find a path that helps you regain a sense of ease about the situation in which you have found yourself and the way the world looks to you now. This is not a guidebook about treatment options and will not give any medical advice. We list places where you can find further information at the end of the book in the appendix. Your doctor who knows your medical circumstances is always your first port of call.

This book is about suggesting different perspectives on where you are now, where you would like to be as you move forward in your cancer journey, and proven strategies that might help you get there. You may even find these techniques helpful in other aspects of your life and should feel free to apply them if you think they seem to be relevant. The book is structured so that each chapter works on its own. You can choose what part seems most relevant to you now. However, the chapters do all build on each other, so it may be helpful to start at the beginning and work your way through to the end. I include personal stories from different men and women who have been in a similar situation to you and hope you will find this both comforting and inspiring. Everyone's experience of prostate cancer is their own, and there is no one right or wrong way to approach this. However, there is nothing quite like personal experience and the wisdom that comes from this experience. In the final chapter of this book, I talk about the idea of survivorship and how you can build a survivorship plan for yourself to help you move forward with confidence and strength.

Note that in this book I use the word '**partner**' to refer to male and female spouses or intimate partners, and also to close friends.

Why do I feel like this?

A common way to explain why the experience of cancer causes feelings of anxiety or sadness is to describe it as a *major life stress*. A major life stress is when an event happens to us that causes threat or danger to things that matter to us most. Cancer is a threat that goes to the core of us. It is first and foremost a threat to life and survival, and many people report that the first question they asked their doctor after hearing the news was: 'Will this cancer kill me?'

Cancer can also be a threat to a person's sense of self: 'Will I be the same as I was before or will I be changed? Less me in some way? Will I still be able to do the things that matter to me?' Cancer can threaten a person's relationships: 'Will I still be loved and cared for? Will people want to be close to me?'

So, no surprises then, that a diagnosis of cancer is often (almost always) accompanied by feelings of fear, shock ('I never heard a word after I heard him say it was cancer!'), anger, deep sadness and confusion. You might have found it hard to concentrate, and had physical signs of stress such as an upset stomach, feeling on edge or irritable, or had restless sleep. Perhaps you find yourself still feeling this way, some or a lot of the time.

A way of explaining why this happens is to think of what would happen if you were facing a tiger! We are all organisms made to recognise threats and respond in a way that will protect ourselves from harm. So, if you were a hunter (or a gatherer) and you found yourself faced by a tiger, your body would instantly recognise the tiger as a serious threat to life and wellbeing and would get you ready biologically to fight or to run (the 'fight or flight' response). Your body does this through an immediate hormonal reaction where your adrenal glands (on top of your kidneys) pump out adrenalin and noradrenalin, and these internal chemicals make your heart go faster, your mouth feels dry, your pupils dilate, and your gut stop working (among a few other things), you become poised to respond to the tiger in front of you. And while that's all quite helpful in the face of an actual tiger, it's not so helpful when the threat is cancer. Instead, right when you are thinking about and trying to rationally work out what the cancer diagnosis means for you and what next steps you need to take, your body is sending out physical fear reactions, and the emotions that go with this are inevitably unpleasant, such as feeling sad, anxious, or afraid.

The very good news is that you can do something about this. There are skills and strategies you can learn to help you meet the problems cancer brings and better manage both physical and emotional challenges. That is what this book is about, explaining ways to moderate or manage psychological and coping responses to cancer in order to live your life fully, the way that you wish.

An important point to make here is that cancer is not just one experience. It is a journey marked by different hurdles. The first hurdle is the diagnosis itself, learning about the extent and nature of the cancer and what treatment options are possible. As a time of uncertainty and distress, this one heads the list. Once a decision about treatment is made, a feeling of calm may come, at least until the preparation for and time of treatment, and then it is 'action stations' again. Recovering from treatment can also be tough, especially learning how to manage any treatment side effects, such as urinary continence, erectile dysfunction, or bowel problems. Medical check-ups can be stressful, especially PSA test time (sometimes unhelpfully called *PSA-itis*). In the longer term, the issue that many men and their partners find most challenging is coping with sexual changes. Our sexual self is a big part of who we are and an important part of many relationships, so changes in this area can be devastating. Acknowledging the aspects of prostate cancer that are most hard and the loss and changes prostate cancer may have brought to your life is part of healing and allows you to make choices about how to move forward.

How do I move forward?

As you progress though this book I ask you to reflect on your experiences, your strengths, what works well for you, and some of the ways you might not serve yourself well. I want you to become your own best friend. A journal or notebook to jot down your thoughts and reflections will help you in this process and will mark the changes as you go along.

You will also see in each chapter an **Activity** section with practical questions and tasks for you to do. These are based on my experiences of working with men and their partners from all sorts of backgrounds. They can be very helpful to your journey in dealing with cancer and I strongly recommend that you take the time when ready to read and undertake these activities.

Activity

As a first step, think about how you felt when you first found out about the cancer and see if you can recall the thoughts that ran through your mind. Did you have one strong worry or a stream of concerns that rapidly replaced each other? Was there one strong emotion you felt? How did your body respond physically? What was your first coping reaction? Did you look for a cave for comfort or did you come out fighting? Taking some time to sit with these feelings and thoughts will help you to increase your awareness of what the diagnosis means to you. This might be uncomfortable, but awareness is the first step to understanding your response, your strengths, and your challenge points.

Next, draw a map on a piece of paper with four circles, one for thoughts, one for emotions, one for physical reactions and one for actions. Fill in examples in each box of what sort of thoughts, emotions, physical reactions and actions you remember feeling and doing. What actions did you take that were helpful? What did not work so well? Now think back to a different example in your life when you have had a difficult time, perhaps a job loss, serious illness in someone you cared for, the death of a loved one, the end of a relationship. Were your feelings then similar to now, or different? Do you have a typical way of coping with stress, and how well does this serve you?

Personal Stories

Reading personal stories from other survivors can help you to reflect more deeply on your own experience; can give you new ideas about how to manage difficulties as they arise; inspire you about what is possible after cancer; and help you feel less alone in your experience. You might like to think about how these stories are similar or different to your personal story. Remember, everyone is different and there is no single right or wrong way to cope. Below are personal stories from David and Pam about their experiences with prostate cancer, the challenges they faced, and how they overcame these. They share with us how the knowledge they gained from their own experience helped them to support their son when he was later diagnosed with prostate cancer at the young age of 42 years. Gary talks about his experience from the perspective of a gay man and how he chose to face his cancer from a position of strength.

David

I was working at Zurich Financial Services when I went along for the usual executive health check. Following the full check-up, which included a PSA blood test and a digital rectal examination (DRE), I was told to see a urologist immediately. He performed a biopsy and confirmed I had cancer.

For anyone to be told this, it's a big shock. One of the dilemmas for me was whether to be open with my staff and friends. I'm open by nature, so I went back to the office and with a bit of difficulty told the people closest to me the verdict. The next weekend I informed my closest friends. That sent shockwaves through people of my own age group. I was 51 then. Many friends and colleagues of my age underwent similar tests and one of them was in hospital weeks later for heart bypass surgery.

Treatment options for prostate cancer depend on your age and the severity of the cancer. Because I was relatively young, 50 years old, and had no symptoms, a radical prostatectomy was a real option for me as the urologist was confident I had a cancer that was confined to the prostate.

Treatment options for prostate cancer can result in incontinence and impotence. The medical professionals try for the trifecta: to get rid of the cancer and have good continence and erectile function. After surgery I was incontinent for a while. That was soon overcome with pelvic floor exercises, but the operation rendered me impotent. Over the years erectile function did come back but not enough for penetration, so my wife Pam and I have had to try other methods. Initially I tried oral medications — that didn't work and then injection therapy but suffered great pain with a chemical reaction. The vacuum device was our next option, and our relationship and sex life was as good as it had ever been. However, it was a tedious process at first. Six and a half years ago I put my reluctance for another operation to one side and had a penile prosthesis implanted. I can now faithfully report that after 45 years of marriage our 'love making' could not be better.

I'm now in my sixteenth year since my radical prostatectomy. I do realise someday the cancer may come back and I'm prepared for that. Prostate cancer is something I wouldn't wish on my worst enemy but having been through the experience Pam and I now appreciate life to the fullest extent. Family, friends and my business network are all very important to me and I work hard to maximise my opportunities, endeavouring to make a difference every day. These days I'm working hard on raising awareness and making it easier for those diagnosed with prostate cancer, their carers and family. I'm National Chairman of Prostate Cancer Foundation of Australia (PCFA) and together with Pam, we lead the Sydney Adventist Hospital — Prostate Cancer Support Group. PCFA now has affiliated Prostate Cancer Support Groups across Australia in every state and territory. I'm an advocate for regular checks and talking to your doctor about men's health generally, especially for those 50 or over. Us blokes need to wake up and take our health seriously.

You would not wish prostate cancer on your worst enemy, but the challenging experience Pam and I faced as a loving couple has enriched our lives.

Pam

Just hearing the word 'cancer' means emotional turmoil. We were no different. Like a lot of men, David thought himself fairly bulletproof, and it was with some reluctance and the insistence of the CEO of Zurich Financial Services that all the executives underwent a full medical check. David was the first to report a problem! When he announced the results, the news sent shock waves amongst his colleagues and friends in the insurance industry. Our family and friends were also stunned.

David had no idea if there was any family medical history that could have rung alarm bells previously.

After a long consult with our urologist that confirmed cancer we left his rooms trying to make sense of how, why and what next needed to be done to get our thought processes working properly and how to best 'attack' what lay ahead. David is of the opinion that most things can be overcome, and life can be made easier by being well organised. We elected to start by making yet another long list.

This included questions for our GP, a consult with a radiation oncologist and foremost, letting our teenage children know of the outcome. The burning question of 'who do you tell', beyond immediate family, and should work colleagues be included, was quickly decided as David is a very open person. We were upfront and let everyone know.

The list of those important items to be looked at included attending to financial papers, our wills, and David's work situation. We weren't surprised when some people found it difficult and uncomfortable to talk over the diagnosis with us.

Coping with the cancer diagnosis included wondering what the end result would be and learning more about the prostate and its function. Do we really need it? Can we live without it? How will the treatment affect our relationship?

We quickly learnt that only about 10 % of what the medical professional is telling you will sink in. Hopefully, that person (and other consultants) will give you some written information to take away, whether it is notes used in describing your biopsy results or more importantly, diagrams of your anatomy with informative booklets and leaflets on the subject. We certainly found it of great benefit to both be included in the consultations. Two sets of ears mean you'll remember more. After all, if you are in a relationship, it is very much a couples' issue.

The emotional turmoil includes anger, denial, confusion and frustration. Here we were at 50 and 51, 'in the prime of our lives' and we were confronted with cancer which we thought was 'an old man's disease'. Before all this happened, we did not even know how to pronounce 'prostate' cancer let alone understand that the implications were. What a learning curve!

It was important to understand the treatment options available but as some of the newer options weren't around, ours included doing nothing (watchful waiting as it was then called), a radical prostatectomy (surgery), or external beam radiation therapy. In David's case, all agreed that surgery was his best bet of ridding himself of the cancer and David still states that if he had his time over he'd proceed with this choice. And I agree. It's of little benefit to suddenly have tunnel vision whether you're the patient or the carer. Communication during this time is paramount. Women share personal experiences with other women. We ask questions, seek information and manage health issues and are proactive in undergoing tests. We want men to become the same. Our close friends rallied to discuss the choices, read up on the disease, understand our situation and gave us the added confidence that we were making the right choice. It helped that one of these friends has a long history with breast cancer.

Thankfully too, our urologist had a great 'game plan' in that he used his patients to telephone counsel newly diagnosed men. What a relief it was to have the lovely voice of a fellow patient speaking to David and to give him confidence about the road ahead. Friends and colleagues who had undergone this type of surgery soon rallied when they heard the news. It was a 'security blanket' we couldn't have done without as any little hitch in the process of recovery was dealt with by a simple phone call.

David was a great patient, which I was surprised about! His recovery went according to plan. Each day was different — emotions soared, rest and recuperation were well monitored and on occasions visitors and phone calls were restricted by me. We appreciated everyone's concerns. By the time he was ready to return to the office he'd overcome his incontinence with pelvic floor exercises, but the ongoing issue of erectile dysfunction was another learning curve.

As a seasoned carer of parents and elderly relatives, I made sure I was eating well, taking time out and getting some exercise — probably not enough. Still, under the circumstances, apart from the emotional rollercoaster, I survived. Communicating with those nearest and dearest to me gave me the ultimate support I needed!

Postscript June 2020 — David & Pam

Our journey continues, and fortunately, at 75 and 73, we are in good health with a second penile implant. We are enjoying life to the full, albeit with another prostate cancer case in our immediate family. We have always said we would be ready for any eventuality, especially as it relates to prostate cancer and it is just as well as Mark, our youngest son, was diagnosed with the disease in November 2019. We knew only too well that prostate cancer can have a genetic factor. With that in mind, our two sons Scott 46 and Mark 42, have had full medicals annually since they were 40, which includes the PSA blood test and the digital rectal examination. Once again, early detection has been a key factor with Mark's diagnosis thanks to a diligent GP and then the surgical option by a talented urologist. Mark had a robotic-assisted radical prostatectomy in December 2019 and he has recovered well to hopefully become another family survivor of this disease. His urologist is confident the cancer was confined to the capsule, and Mark has full continence and erectile function which is a great relief to him and his wife Lucie and all of us. He is now undergoing DNA testing to ascertain if there is a gene fault that has not yet been established in the family.

We are now even more convinced that annual medical examinations are very important for all those over 50 as early detection is key for cancer, serious illnesses and diseases. This is especially so for those families with medical histories of cancer and other illnesses and diseases. As in our family's case, age 40 is the recommended benchmark.

We are indeed a very fortunate couple.

Gary

I guess when I look back over my life, I have seen a lot of cancer. My mother died of breast cancer when I was seventeen and just starting university. My father died of cancer when he was 60 years old. He was of that stoic age where he never spoke about his cancer and it was a short and rapid illness. I am fairly sure that he had prostate cancer, and my mother dying at such a young age pretty much was the end of him. So as a result, I was always very health-conscious and consistent with getting regular health checks and tests. I started having PSA tests when I was 45 years old, and when my PSA started to move around a bit my GP referred me to a specialist urologist who kept a close eye on me. But even though I knew I had this risk, I still was not prepared when I got the call to say something was wrong. I remember I was at Woolworths buying my vegetables when my doctor called me. I went straight into shock and walked out without paying and so had to go back later. That weekend I just went into hibernation and spoke to no one. I spent the whole weekend with 'Dr. Google' finding everything I could online about prostate cancer, looking for options and trying to make sense of it all. That weekend I came to see I had a choice. I could spiral into depression, or I could fight it. So, I came to accept the situation and decided to take control. I had a lot to live for both from a career perspective and personally. I was single and so had to rely on myself. But I did have friends, so I contacted all my friends and workmates to share the news about what had happened and what I was going to do about it. This helped me feel more in control. Two weeks later, my doctor laid all the options on the table for me. I chose to have robotic surgery. With my family history, I just wanted it out. Having said that, today, given the advances stemming from research, etcetera, my advice is to think carefully about your options and take your time.

I did well after surgery, was out of hospital quickly and back to work in five weeks. That was too quick though. I should have taken more time as I got a bit rundown. I think I wanted to see myself as progressing fast, and getting back to work was part of that picture for me. Incontinence settled down within about a month and I did get my erections back within six months. And I am here. I am alive. For me, it is a success story.

I do feel that being a gay man has made me very resilient. I thought I had been through worse in my life, and as I said above, I have a lot to live for. I have always liked change, in work and where I live, and in so many other ways, so I am good at reinventing myself, and you do need to reinvent yourself after prostate cancer. I see myself as a survivor. For many men, whether you are gay or straight, it is the sex side of things that worries you the most at first and causes anxiety. Whatever your situation, you need to reinvent yourself, certainly when it comes to sex. And the shock and despair you experience, the same applies. Reinvention is the key — an ability to change.

Not being able to 'cum' is a big deal for many gay men. Not so much for me. I think sex is about the journey more than the 'happy ending'. When you think about it, we are taught as we grow up about sex, but not about love and relationships. You do worry about it as a single person, but I have never been rejected as a partner because of my cancer. Early on, I worried that I would never get another partner and maybe never have sex again. But that is not what happened. I do not share my cancer situation with every man I meet, not unless it looks like it is going to be an ongoing relationship. Many men are surprised to hear you can still orgasm but not 'cum'. I say, 'I am doing my bit for the 'green' movement by cutting down on washing my sheets and saving water!'. Today, I co-lead a support group for gay men with cancer, and I often say, gentlemen, you need to be honest with yourself and work at this. You need to learn how to love again. I also say breathe. The cancer is not going to kill you tomorrow. Get informed and plan, take action but do not overdo it. Give yourself time to adjust and then heal.

As you can see, I chose to face my cancer from a position of strength. My cancer story is not a story of sorrow. It is a story of survival.

Chapter 2

'Why me?' On Being Diagnosed With Prostate Cancer

Before going any further, it is important to remember that individuals differ. This seems like a simple statement that we all know and agree with, but we often operate in the world as if everyone thinks and acts as we do, and if they don't, they should. While some people may react to life a lot like you, mostly they won't, and this includes people close to you. Accepting this upfront can help prevent misunderstanding. Accepting your own reaction to being diagnosed with prostate cancer as just that — your own — is crucial. In other words, guard against judging yourself (or others) and give yourself a break!

The things that influence how a person reacts to a cancer diagnosis include age, gender, educational background, and previous life experiences. We know this from relentless research in the field, however it just makes sense if you think it through. For example, younger men often report higher levels of distress than older men. This may relate to the stage of life younger men are at, perhaps still raising children, building a career, not being financially well established and certainly not expecting a cancer diagnosis at this age. Some younger men with prostate cancer may not yet have had children or are hoping for more children and so face the potential loss of fertility. Perhaps their intimate relationship is new and not yet well established, or they do not have a partner and fear that now it will be even harder to form a relationship. Younger men may find they feel different from their peers and become isolated from their usual supports.

For older men, the issues may be different. Older men may finally have retired from the full-time workforce and be gearing up to enjoy a different pace of life and to doing the things they have long dreamed about, like a 'grey nomad' holiday, playing more golf, or spending time with grandchildren. Older men may be facing other health problems as well, such as heart disease or arthritis, and these things can make it harder to manage the physical issues associated with prostate cancer and its treatment. Older men who are not partnered may find they feel alone, and might now find it harder to connect with new partners or their usual networks or feel nervous about how people will react to them.

What does cancer mean to me?

Previous personal experience with cancer also has an impact on how a man reacts to a cancer diagnosis. A man has a higher chance of being diagnosed with prostate cancer if he has a first-degree relative (a father or brother) who has had prostate cancer. If your relative had a difficult time with prostate cancer and perhaps did not do well after treatment, this will influence your expectations and fears about what might happen to you. Beyond this, as we age, it is almost impossible not to have friends or relatives with cancer given that older age is a risk factor for the most common cancers such as breast, colorectal and prostate cancer. Whatever the nature of the cancer experiences we have observed, we can't help but weave this into our internal or mental picture of what having cancer means. If you have known people who managed well after cancer, you may see your prostate cancer as a challenge that you can overcome. However, if your personal experiences of cancer have been mostly negative, your prostate cancer may seem like a giant looming threat.

Why does this matter? Having cancer can feel overwhelming and confusing. If you can gain some understanding of what lies underneath or directs your strongest reactions, you will be better able to manage your response in a way that works more effectively for you. For example, if you are clear about which of your life goals are most threatened by the cancer, you can direct efforts to plan how you might still achieve those goals, but in a different way. If you had a very negative personal cancer experience in the past that is influencing how you are responding now, you can challenge the actual relevance of this past experience to your current situation. Getting clear about your life goals and what cancer means to you is important in making sense of where you are right now.

Being a Man and Coping with Cancer

What also matters is understanding your own personal coping style. Most of us have our own typical approaches to problems or challenges. A lot of this is learnt in our childhood by what our parents and our peer group tell us, and what they model by their own behaviour. It is fair to say that boys are taught or expected to be strong and fearless. If you break this approach down to what it means in terms of behaviour, you could reasonably list: don't cry when you are hurt; keep your feelings to yourself; take risks; fight back; be self-reliant; and if it is broken, just fix it! These strategies are often described as male stoicism: the 'hang tough' and 'be a man' approach — recognise any of this? As a result, compared to women, men seek preventative health care services less often; are less likely to report depression but more likely to commit suicide, and are much less likely to use cancer support services. In brief, many blokes approach their health in ways that are just not that helpful; that make it tougher for themselves in the short and long term; and that to their detriment, bottle up difficult emotions and block support.

In my own research on masculinity and men with prostate cancer, we identified five different aspects of masculinity that men felt were important in understanding how prostate cancer affected their lives and also how they coped. These were optimistic action, sexual importance, family responsibilities, emotional self-reliance and strength and fitness. Optimistic action referred to an action-oriented approach to dealing with problems, for example, always looking for the good in a situation or taking action in the face of problems. Emotional self-reliance was about keeping your feelings to yourself or tending not to talk about your worries. Strength and fitness was about being physically strong and an active person. Sexual importance was about being able to have an erection and have sex. Family responsibilities covered looking after your partner or family. All of these things were important to men to varying degrees, depending on their life circumstances. The key here is to be aware of the extent to which these aspects matter to you to help you get a sense of how your diagnosis might be affecting your perspective on life in the future. This chapter is not about necessarily changing these perspectives but more about understanding yourself and being prepared to be flexible.

The key is to decide, in the face of a prostate cancer diagnosis, to adopt strategies that help you rather than hinder you. A helpful analogy here is to think about coping strategies as tools in your toolbox. You would not try to change a tyre using an everyday shifting spanner or wrench unless you wanted to make things really hard for yourself. When you work on a car you have a box full of tools where each tool works differently for different parts of the engine and chassis. In coping with cancer you might have one tool you prefer the most, but if it doesn't seem to be working or getting you the results you want, then another tool might make things a lot easier.

Coping approaches or tools are often put into two broad groups: problem-solving or emotion-focused. *Problem-solving coping* is just that — applying strategies to solve the problem. The aim is to fix it. In the case of a prostate cancer diagnosis, this might mean seeking different medical opinions, looking up medical information on the Internet, making a decision, and having treatment. Problem-solving is an active approach that achieves outcomes and helps you to move forward in a practical and tangible way.

Emotion-focused coping applies strategies to reduce painful or difficult emotions or feelings of distress. This can include talking to other people about how you feel, crying or expressing emotion, and using stress management and relaxation techniques. These strategies are useful in keeping an even keel and managing how you feel while going through the cancer, and are a natural complement to problem-solving.

Avoiding thinking (or talking) about the cancer is another type of emotion-focused coping that can be helpful in some situations, and not so helpful in others. For example, if you are about to have a biopsy or a painful medical procedure, not thinking about this and instead imagining you are on a beach in Fiji might be very helpful as a short-term distraction. However, imagining you are in Fiji all or most of the time will likely hinder your ability to make decisions and communicate with others close to you about what is happening in your life.

The trick then is to use flexible coping, being prepared to change tack if your current approach is not working and being open to possibilities and change. In brief, you want a toolbox that will help you get the best outcome you can for yourself and for those close to you.

What are the likely issues I will face in the future?

Over time, most men find that the difficult feelings they experience when they are diagnosed with prostate cancer ease. Life starts to return to normal (although many say a 'different normal') and unless a specific issue comes up, such as a PSA blood test or a health complication, they feel life is just as good as it was before the cancer. The most persistent long-term problem for men is usually on the sexual side of things. Most prostate cancer treatments lead to changes in sexual function, for example, being unable to get an erection or an erection not as firm as before treatment, and a loss of sexual desire. For men, this can have a deep effect on how they see themselves as a man. Many men have told me they feel less vital as a result of these sexual changes and that getting themselves back to feeling masculine and confident with sex and relationships has been difficult, and for many is still a 'work in progress'.

Other worries can include ongoing tiredness, and this may be a result of treatment or the stress associated with the whole cancer experience. Tiredness can make it difficult to get back to usual activities and the things that you enjoy. While treatment effects on urinary and bowel function often resolve in the short- to medium-term, coping with these in the meantime requires planning and effort. If a man is having hormone-blocking treatment this can lead to tiredness, a low mood, loss of muscle strength and poorer mental concentration. Strategies to maintain wellbeing are crucial.

For many men, a feeling of uncertainty about the future and whether the cancer will come back is an ongoing worry. Regardless of the fact that one day we will all die (that is for certain), most of us live as if our days ahead are endless. A diagnosis of cancer means that dying of cancer is a possibility (although again, this is actually true for many of us), and it forces most people to, at least at some level, contemplate their mortality. In this sense the world can appear very different after a diagnosis of prostate cancer — less fair or just — and coming to terms with and accepting a changed understanding of the world and our place in it is a journey all of its own.

Setting Goals

One thing is for sure; if you don't know where you want to go, you probably won't get there! Setting goals is crucial to the approach we suggest in this book. Goals can be short, medium and long term. The trick is for them to be realistic, achievable, important to you, and that you are able to tell when you have got there. A 'small steps' first approach is usually best here.

Activity

For all men at whatever stage of life, prostate cancer threatens their goals and hopes. How has cancer affected your goals and future hopes? Write these down in your own dedicated notebook. Perhaps your goals have changed since the cancer diagnosis and other things have become more important. Looking at your list, which of these matters most to you right now?

Each of your goals will have a different timeline; some might be things you would like to achieve in the short- or medium-term; some might be long-term goals. You might set goals that are about how you are coping with the cancer; or about your relationships and how you would like them to be or to develop. As an example, a short-term goal might be to learn some quick and easy stress reduction strategies, such as deep breathing exercises and a low intensity walking program. As you do this, you can map your overall wellbeing so you can be encouraged by the gains you make. A plan to improve your sexual life might start with short-term goals about pleasant couple activities (such as seeing a movie or going for a dinner 'date') and intimacy, and sensual pleasure, with a medium-term goal to have full sexual intercourse. Long-term goals might be to complete treatment and then go on a long-awaited holiday (best not to wait for 'one day') or to take on a personal physical or mental challenge. You might have long-term life goals you would like to work towards.

What would you like life to look like for you in six or twelve months?

Next, start to list what steps you need to take to achieve these goals? Finally, who can help you with this? Jot down the names of people in your life you could enlist to support, help or encourage you to reach these goals. Talk to someone you trust or who is close to you about your most hoped-for goals. This will help you further clarify and confirm your next steps. Every month or so check back with your list and see how you are going. It is perfectly fine if your list changes, or if new goals come up. The main point of this activity is that you have a sense of direction and that you notice when you achieve goals, and then give yourself a pat on the back!

Now for your toolbox! How do you usually cope with difficulties? What is your main preference and how well does that work for you? Think about a time when you have coped well with a personal challenge and felt very positive about the outcome. How would you describe your approach then? Now think about a time when you were faced with a personal challenge and it did not go so well. How could you have approached this problem differently?

Further on in this book you will find more specific suggestions and ideas about ways to face prostate cancer and to tame the tiger! Feel free to jump ahead, but you might find it helps to do the reflections suggested in this chapter in advance and prioritise your goals.

Personal Stories

Below is a personal story from Peter about his experience with prostate cancer at a young age, the difficulties he faced after surgery, and the strategies he used to move forward. Your experience may be similar in some ways to Peters' story or very different. A fairly common element though that men do report is feeling you are alone, and as Peter's story shows, this need not be the case.

Peter

> When I was diagnosed with prostate cancer at the age of 52, (in 1996), after a routine blood test (PSA), the shock was enormous. At the time, such was the neglected state of awareness of men's health issues, I didn't even know what my prostate was — or, for that matter, what it did. As well, as a health professional — a physiotherapist — for the previous twenty years, I had followed a lifestyle of exercise, diet and meditation, one which the gurus had promised would significantly lessen the risk of cardiac disease and cancer. Not completely true, I found.
>
> To add to the shock, virtually any invasive treatment I could undertake had the potential of being nasty. To me, at the time, surgery (radical prostatectomy) seemed to offer the best chance for survival. At this stage, some sixteen years later, it certainly appears to have achieved that — something for which I am decidedly grateful.
>
> However, after the prostatectomy in February 1996, I was left severely incontinent, to the extent where I was filling six incontinence pads a day during the first six months. I found that this was seriously impacting my lifestyle, as well as my professional career, emotional health, exercise activity, sex life and relationships. In fact, I was also suffering from erectile dysfunction, a situation in itself I was not coping with. I became very despondent and

developed reactive depression. Worse still, I could find no other men who had been through this process. I felt very isolated. In my mind, I was the only man in the world in this situation.

The frustration, anger — and indeed, often rage — I felt led me to resolve to change things. The alternative was to accept a seriously reduced lifestyle. In fact, suicide appeared an attractive proposition. The vulnerable time was driving home from work — tired, leaking and feeling devastated that lovemaking may never be a reality again. I really was feeling hopeless and despairing.

It was then that a quiet voice deep inside took command and ordered me to quell my panic — to be calm. In desperation, I sought out some physiotherapy colleagues who I knew treated women with incontinence. They taught me how to execute standard pelvic floor muscles exercises, which I performed aggressively and with enormous motivation. The action began to stem the flow, and after some months, I had controlled the loss to about a dozen leakages a day. While this was more acceptable and manageable in terms of my lifestyle, I still found that just one leakage would trigger a depression cycle, one of the now obvious psychosocial legacies resulting from my choice of treatment.

At this stage, I put an advertisement in the local paper and formed the first Prostate Cancer Support Group in Queensland. From this, I hoped to find some answers to assist both me and the many others I soon found who were fellow sufferers. (With the assistance of Cancer Council Queensland, the Brisbane Prostate Cancer Support Group is now one of the largest groups in the country, and we have joined with other groups nationally as part of Prostate Cancer Foundation of Australia. No man need be alone again!)

I then worked to improve my incontinence to another level. Some four years after diagnosis, I designed an intensive exercise program aiming to develop a highly efficient (super fit) neuromuscular and vascular system which controls and supplies all the structures that form the pelvic and abdominal cavities. The idea was to increase the local and collateral pelvic circulation. For me, that meant endurance-type exercise — running, cycling, and gym. As well, I wanted to retrain elements of the neural reflex circuitry of all the muscles and sphincters which control continence. I did this with jogging, firstly on flat ground, then uneven ground, then uphills, harder and faster. Finally, I worked on integrating pelvic floor muscle activity with abdominal muscle activity. This meant contracting the pelvic floor muscles and the abdominal muscles simultaneously while functionally doing 'crunches'.

After some six months of this program, the leakage diminished to maybe a few drops every few days. This was something I could live with. But the best result was that it also broke the depression cycle.

In the meantime, I had learned to rehabilitate my erectile dysfunction with prostaglandin injections. The final aspect of coming to terms with this sort of diagnosis and treatment was to confront and understand the process of grief and loss. We need to know of the four main stages of grief — denial, anger, depression and acceptance. That way, we can learn to accept the new reality of our life.

Adjustment often requires time and re-evaluation of what it means to be a male; it may challenge our belief systems and values, one's faith and the very purpose of being. My aim was to really live a meaningful and contented life. For me, this enlightenment is one of the 'gifts' that a life-threatening condition can reveal.

Chapter 3

'Me too!' On Loving Someone With Prostate Cancer

When cancer happens in a family, all thoughts go first to the needs and worries of the person who has the cancer. However, in many cases, the partners of men with prostate cancer report more distress and worry than do the men themselves. It is hard to know for sure why this is so, and of course all couples will have their own habits of coping and ways of facing challenges. However, it can be the case that watching your partner go through the experience of cancer can seem harder than actually having it. Partners sit inside of the cancer survivorship experience and can be seen themselves as 'cancer survivors'.

Standing beside someone you love and watching them undergo painful or difficult procedures and face a threat to their life is heartbreaking. You might feel powerless to help. You might not really understand or know what the cancer diagnosis actually means, particularly if you haven't been involved in the doctor's visits or if you haven't discussed this as a couple. If your partner has become withdrawn then you might feel very alone and frustrated in all of this.

Perhaps you feel you are not able to reach out for help — after all, you don't have cancer! Many partners have told me that they have felt guilty for wanting support for themselves. You might be the one who takes care of the family's health, and perhaps you tend to put yourself last when it comes to care and attention.

Finally, often in relationships there is one person who is the 'emotional barometer' and who picks up on negative emotion first and takes on the job of easing the tension. If this is you, then that is a very big job, and it is exhausting!

Partners often report different worries than the patient, and it can be hard to share these when you see your job as being a support person. In my own work, some partners have told me about worrying how they will manage if the man they are with dies, especially if they have been together for many years. That is a hard fear to share. You might be worried about how you are managing financially now, and what the future might bring, but feel unable to discuss this. You might also fear what being alone might be like, and be fearful of becoming isolated and unsupported in your own life challenges.

You may have found that in the early phase of the illness, you were well supported by friends and family, but that over time you are expected to just 'get on with it'. The experience of prostate cancer is, for most, a long journey, with ongoing tests and medical checks. So even though treatment might be over, the worry can remain.

Coping with treatment side effects can be tough for you too. It might mean that you don't go out as often or see friends as much as you used to. Your sex life will be affected as well, and you might be feeling a loss of closeness and physical touch. This might be making you start to feel uncertain about your own attractiveness as a sexual mate.

If the man has experienced a cancer recurrence and is on hormonal blocking medication, there may be stress associated with balancing treatment side effects, quality of life, and controlling the cancer. To say this can be an emotional roller coaster is an understatement.

Looking After Yourself

The first lesson you need to learn and accept is that you matter. Your own wellbeing and mental health remain important for you, as a unique and valuable person in this world. (Yes, this is a lecture just for you!) You also matter for the man who relies on your support, so if you feel you can't look after yourself just for you, then do it for him!

If you are coping well, there will be a likely positive flow-on effect to those around you, so make yourself a priority. This might mean scheduling time to do things you find pleasurable, keeping up with your friends, and making time for hobbies and interests.

You also have a right to discuss how you are feeling about the cancer in a private setting with others close to you. This is an important way to seek support that will help you feel less alone and lessen your feelings of distress.

Understanding Coping

In the previous chapter, I talked about the importance of understanding your own personal coping style and taking a flexible approach. Do you have a typical approach to problems? How well does this approach usually work for you?

Remember, we have already talked a little about the two broad groups of coping approaches: problem-solving or emotion-focussed. Problem-solving applies strategies to solve the problem. This is an active approach that gets outcomes and helps you to move forward in a practical and tangible way. An example of problem-solving coping as a partner would be to be as informed as you can be about the medical plan. If you are well informed about what the cancer means, what treatments are available, and the likely effects of treatment, then you will feel more confident about being an effective support person. If you are feeling uncertain about what the cancer means, you are more likely to worry and feel sad or anxious about the cancer and the future. Being involved in doctor's visits will help. There is also a lot of easy to find information about prostate cancer on the Internet and through phone helplines, so check the appendix in this book for reliable sources of advice.

Emotion-focused coping helps reduce unpleasant emotions. For some people this means talking to their friends or close family members about what is going on and how they feel. (Some of us rehearsed this as teenagers and young adults with endless telephone conversations with our friends!) A good cry can help as well. Emotion-focused coping is important and balances and complements problem-solving coping.

As described earlier, avoiding thinking (or talking) about the cancer is another type of emotion-focused coping that is often not so helpful, especially for you as a partner and support person. If you avoid a painful issue, it gets stronger as a worry — the more you push it away, the stronger it will come back. By avoiding a painful problem, we can give it more power to hurt us.

Activity

When cancer hits a couple, it affects goals in life for both of them. It can seem like a roadblock to long hoped for plans or can make past hopes seem not as important. This can leave you feeling like you have lost control of the ship! Reconnecting with goals and being clear about where you are heading is crucial.

Think about how prostate cancer has affected ***your*** future goals and hopes. Have your goals changed (or been forgotten) since your partner was diagnosed with cancer? What are the things that matter to you most now in the short-term? Do you have medium- or long-term goals? Perhaps you have lost sight of these in the face of the stress of the cancer and looking after your mate. If so, now is a great time to remember the things that are important to you and, if needed, set new goals.

You might set goals that are about looking after yourself right now. You might have longer-term life goals you would like to renew and work towards. What would life look like for you in six or twelve months' time in the best of worlds? Write down a list of goals for right now, and for in six months, and for in a year or two. What steps do you need to take to achieve these goals, and who can help you with these?

Talk to someone you trust about your most important goals. This will help you confirm your agreement to look after yourself as you deserve. Check your list regularly to see how you are going and revise or change your goals if needed. Again, the main point of this activity is that you have a sense of where you are headed and that you start to place a priority on your own wellbeing and life happiness without feeling guilty about it.

Now think about how you usually cope with difficulties? What is your main style of coping and how well is this working for you now? Think about a time when you have coped well with a difficult problem and felt pleased with how it turned out. How would you describe your approach then? Now think about a time when you were faced with a problem, and it did not go so well. How could you have approached this differently? Are there new coping skills you might need to learn?

Further on in this book, you will find more specific advice about ways to look after yourself and to nurture your relationship with your partner. Feel free to move ahead to chapters that interest you. It will help though if you take the time to reflect on your goals as suggested in this chapter and be clear about where you would like to head.

Personal Stories

Below are personal stories from Avryl and Carole about their experiences when their partners were diagnosed with prostate cancer and the challenges they faced walking the path with them.

Avryl

My husband had a radical prostatectomy in 2009, so it is a few years down the track for me at present, though I still get upset thinking about it even now. I think it was just such a total shock. I was quite young at the time, only 48, and we never saw this coming. I think Graham was very numb when it happened. I played the strong person that I am, but I couldn't help thinking: 'Is he going to die? Am I going to lose him?' It is our second marriage, and we feel we are very lucky that we found each other the second time around. We have a very special bond. Graham is a very special person with a beautiful heart and good values. So when this happened I thought: 'Why him?' It seemed so unfair.

As a woman, I think you do want your man to be the strong one to take care of you, and then all of a sudden your world is being turned upside down. Definitely, I felt alone and that I couldn't talk to anyone. I didn't think anyone could understand how I was feeling. As well, no one really knew what we were going through because it was all very personal, so we kept a lot of it to ourselves. After his operation, we just thought he would be back to normal, so to speak. We didn't get any information to prepare us to deal with his incontinence, or his erectile problems. We had no idea really about what was ahead of us.

After the operation, Graham was incontinent and wearing pads. He felt dirty and not a man anymore, even though I said it didn't worry me. He didn't want to touch me because of how he was feeling, we weren't having sex anymore, and I felt unloved and alone. All the romance had gone and we were just living together, almost like we were brother and sister. I was annoying him; maybe we were annoying each other, and we were arguing where we never used to argue, over the stupidest things.

I threw myself into work; it was a way of trying to run away from it all. About twelve months after his surgery I had an anxiety attack at work. I had never had one before and thought I was having a heart attack! It was almost like once he was on the mend, I collapsed. I think it was just my body coping with all that was happening. I tend to be like that at times, very strong, on the go, coping with anything that comes along with the biggest of shoulders and then when I stop, I just collapse in a heap. I had always felt guilty thinking about me and my needs because it wasn't about me; it was about him. He was the one with the cancer. I'm lucky to have close girlfriends to have some fun with and turn off, but I didn't really talk to them about it. Sometimes I would just burst into tears, and then I would feel like an idiot because I couldn't explain what I was crying about. It was just me letting my emotions go.

Now, I think we have grown as a couple. I think it shows we can face anything. I know our relationship has always been strong, but now it's stronger than ever. However, I wouldn't want anyone else to have to go through this.

My main message to partners is to look for support and feel comfortable to talk and seek help. Going to a support group and getting help from people who know what you are going through makes all the difference. For me, talking to another woman who has been through this was a huge support and relief. The more you talk about it, the more you see that there are other people in the same situation as you, and you are able to find hope that you will get through it.

Carole

David was diagnosed with prostate cancer in 1999, and it was traumatic for both of us. He was anxious, and his way of dealing with it, at least at first, was to search for alternatives and talk to a lot of people, but not to me. That left me feeling left out and angry. Finally, he had his treatment, radical prostatectomy, and then we had his treatment side effects to deal with. It really was a very tough time for him, and for me.

I think I felt lost, totally lost. I remember thinking, 'I can't do this'. Looking back, I don't think we got very good support from the medical team. I think David kept the physical problems he was struggling with to himself a lot, and we didn't have a good support network around us. It was a second marriage for both of us, so I felt I couldn't talk to the family. I didn't really have anyone I felt I could talk to about it.

I learnt a lot from this experience, about compassion and about caring for others, listening to their stories and then trying to find out where they can get help. I have learnt to look after myself. To help myself relax I put music on to listen to late at night because I am not the best sleeper, and this helps me wind down. I work, I keep active and listen to the radio every day. It is a distraction from worry, and I learn new things about the world all the time.

I think that partners should be involved in the doctors' consultations so everyone is on the same page. I also think we need to have a support service where somebody can talk to couples like David and me because I think there must be lots of people in the exact same situation. As a partner you don't want to take the whole load; you want to share the load. So I guess my advice to couples facing this right now is to talk about it with each other, and if this is hard to do, look for someone to help you talk about it. David and I have talked about all this now, and we are great friends, but I wish we had done this earlier. I think it would have made our journey a lot easier.

Chapter 4

'We're in this together'

A diagnosis of cancer when you are in a couple relationship affects both people in that relationship. And how each individual reacts affects the other. This happens on several levels. First, if your partner is very distressed, then that will be distressing to you. By contrast, if your partner is upset but calm, you might find it easier to be calm as well. It is a two-way street, with each person's reaction having some effect on the other. This does not mean that either of you should hide how you feel. In fact, the opposite is true. It is important to be honest and open about how each of you is feeling. The point is to be aware that although you are both individuals with your own unique approach to things, you are connected emotionally.

On another level — and this is the part you can work on together — how each of you copes will affect the other person's experience and your own. In brief, if people in a couple relationship have a similar approach to coping, they tend to have a smoother run.

As an example, if one person wants to talk about the cancer most of the time and the other person in the relationship prefers to avoid thinking about it until they absolutely have to, this can lead to conflict. Similarly, if for the man his main long term goal is to complete treatment and get back to work whereas his partner wants more of a focus on being together and enjoying each others company, both people may feel frustrated and misunderstood.

Something else to consider is that when you are both under pressure (and a prostate cancer diagnosis certainly fits that bill!) it can be harder to get on with each other. You might each feel more sensitive and on edge and find that your usual ways of getting over hurdles don't seem to be helping.

It is not that one person is right and the other wrong, just that their individual approaches to the situation are different. It is this difference that can make the journey harder.

So, if no one is right or wrong, what can you do? The key is effective communication. By that, I mean communication that allows each person to have a say and feel heard, with both of you working together as a team. What is also important is remembering that you are each under a lot of stress dealing with the cancer, so things that might in the past have been easy to solve can seem tougher. In this situation, putting more effort into how you communicate with each other can make all the difference.

Communicating Effectively With Your Partner

Perhaps the first thing to try and avoid is mind-reading. This goes both ways. In relationships, we often act as if we can read our partners' minds and they can read ours. We think we know why our partner is angry or upset, even though we haven't checked it out with them, and more often than not we think it is all about us. Or we think that our partner should know how we want to be supported and that if they don't give us what we need, then they don't really care or aren't interested.

Compounding the problem, we mind read and then treat our conclusions as if they are fact and react accordingly, even if the trigger issue is actually quite trivial. Who has never thought of their partner: 'If he/she really loved me they would have done the dishes/put out the rubbish/picked up the dry cleaning?'

The first step then is to accept that although you may know your partner better than anyone else in the world, you have never known them under quite these circumstances and that unless you have clairvoyant skills you cannot read their mind. The only way you can know for sure what they are thinking or worrying about is if they let you know. Until you check out your assumptions, they are just your fantasies, not fact.

In reverse then, unless your partner has clairvoyant skills they also cannot read your mind, and expecting them to do so will most likely not get you what you want or need.

So my tip is that first, you need to decide as a couple if you want to work on improving how you communicate. If the answer is 'yes', then you need to agree to work at this together in a non-judgmental and supportive way. By this I mean accepting that you are both unique individuals and that each of you has the right to feel the way you do and that these feelings are not right or wrong — they just are what they are. It is useful to remember here that couples often have quite different ways of coping with problems: one person may tend to want to act and fix things while the other person wants to talk about the issues. This can lead to conflict and feeling alone in the experience.

If you both accept that being different is okay then the next step is to try sharing some of those feelings and talking to each other about what they mean for you. For each of you this might mean first up sharing what your main worry is and how you feel you are coping. Talking this over and then checking with each other to make sure you are both clear about the other person's perspective is central to good communication. You might share how you have been feeling over the past two to three weeks, what thoughts have been worrying you the most, and what seems to help you feel calmer or less stressed.

Once you are clear about where you each are at in terms of your main worries, a good next step might be to check if there are things you can do to help each other cope. Clear and practical suggestions are best. For example, 'if I am upset just hug me and don't try and solve anything' is better than 'just be there for me' or 'if I need to go out to the shed for a while to be on my own, let me have some space but then come down in an hour or so with a cup of tea' is better than 'stop fussing'.

What if talking makes it worse?

Sometimes cancer can feel overwhelming for a couple. This is more likely if the relationship is still new and perhaps not so solid yet, or if you have had troubles in the past. As well, if you have other pressing problems to cope with at the same time, such as money worries or children or ageing parents who need a lot of support from you, the pressure can seem huge.

Getting to the bottom of things without blaming each other for the situation you are in can be challenging. You might need to think back to the things that brought you together in the first place, what it is about each other that you most value, and what are the things now as a couple that bind you together. Are these things still present for you? Are they important? If the answer is 'yes' then reminding yourselves of your shared core values can help you get back a sense of being a team.

Next, remember, the experience of a cancer diagnosis is a major life stress. It doesn't get much tougher than this. So give each other a break and try not to be hard on yourself and your partner. Try and work flexibly on problems and to see each other's points of view. Treat yourself and your partner with kindness.

Finally, if you feel you cannot get on top of this as a couple, seek help. Talking to an experienced, couples-focused psychologist or counsellor can make all the difference.

Activity

Set aside time (about 20 minutes) once or twice each week to talk with each other about how you each are feeling and coping — no problem solving, just listening and making sure you have checked you understand and 'get it'.

The rules are don't judge or criticise and don't interrupt.

Next, think of three to five things your partner could do to support you. Make a commitment to each other to try these out and see how it goes. Be clear about which support action matters the most to each of you.

Be fair.

Finally, take time to do a pleasurable activity with each other that has nothing to do with cancer. By making each other a priority, you will strengthen your feelings of connectedness, and you might even have some fun!

Personal Stories

Below are personal stories from couples who had different challenges and approaches to supporting each other through their prostate cancer experience. Jan and Gordon talk about how weekly meetings helped them keep in touch with what was going on for each other. Jim and Laura found that being patient and accepting each other as they are was crucial. For these couples, taking time to communicate about what was going on became central to their approach in managing the challenges of cancer as a team. Casey talks about how he and his partner worked together as a team and have been able to maintain their intimacy as well as respecting each other's space.

Gordon

I was diagnosed with prostate cancer in early 2004. My PSA was elevated — it was 20 — and after a course of antibiotics it was still going up. The next step was a biopsy that came back positive. Because my PSA was high, radiation therapy seemed a better option than surgery, and so I ended up having high dose brachytherapy, external beam radiation therapy, with a course of hormone treatment that went on for two years after treatment. My PSA stayed down for a couple of years and then started to rise again. As a result, I am now back on hormone treatment and participating in a clinical trial for a new set of drugs. Jan says I rattle with all the pills I am on!

It was pretty rough finding out about the cancer. We came to the point of just accepting I've got cancer and it's not going to go away. We went through a period of having weekly meetings when we would sit down on Saturday mornings and write down what we were going to do, and what were our worries, and things like that. We did this for quite a while.

It is important to work out ways of communicating, because, particularly with men, we are blokes and we don't want to talk about it! But it is necessary to talk about things. Sometimes it is easier to talk to people who are not your spouse or partner. I had a couple of friends that were in the same situation, and we had conversations that I wouldn't have been able to have with Jan at the time. But since then we have been able to work it so that now the conversations that Jan and I have are the same sort of conversations I had with my friends. I think with me, it was getting the confidence to actually say what was on my mind. Partnerships are made by two people trying to work through a system of what happens, and losing a fear that if you say how you feel you might appear to be less a person in your partner's eyes. It is important to be able to actually say this is how I feel or this is the way it is for me at the moment, and have enough trust that it will be seen and supported.

I think part of it is you are brought up to say as boys, particularly of our vintage, that you are the male and you have to be seen as strong and out there.

Jan

When Gordon and I were doing our weekly meetings we would tell our friends. They thought we were mad, but it was really important. We were bogged down; we were a ship without a rudder and didn't know what to do and where to go. Gordon was really lost saying, 'What do I do?

What don't I do?' Making time for good quality honest conversation, even if your list starts off with 'when is the fence going to get repaired?' or 'when is the pool man coming?' or whatever it is, gives you a structure to deal with the 'don't know' stuff that sometimes you don't deal with because it's all too hard.

We do have rows — differences of opinion — but for us, that's about honest discussion and not avoiding the difficult stuff. I don't sit down with Gordon and say, 'Right, we are going to have an honest discussion now'. It's about when the time is right, you sit and say, 'listen there is something we need to have a conversation about'. For me, it's trying to gauge when it's the right time to have that discussion and how far the conversation can go. I think at the end of the day Gordon appreciates the fact that we do put the hard stuff on the table, and this gives him a chance to talk about where he is coming from and how it feels, 'cause he is a bloke, and they tend not to talk about feelings and hopes and goals and aspirations.

Jim

I was diagnosed with prostate cancer in 2007 and was put straight away on hormone therapy, external beam radiation and then high dose brachytherapy. I was on the hormone treatment for over 6 months all told, and that was the worst. I suppose most blokes would say the lack of sex drive was a big concern, but I found it was all the other effects. You start to lose muscle, you don't feel too enthusiastic, you're moody, you end up having some memory loss.

I stopped work immediately, and we had 5 acres at the time and then not long after I decided that we would sell it because Laura wouldn't be able to deal with it. I was getting the property ready for sale, so that occupied my mind a fair bit and gave me something else to think about, but it was pretty tough times. I remember, and I often talk about this, Laura was still teaching and she came home one day and I was sitting out the back on a park bench that we had and she came round the corner of the house and I was sitting there crying my eyes out and she said 'What's wrong with you?' I said 'I need a dog. I am sitting here by myself, no one to talk to, you are off at work, and I am feeling miserable.' So we ended up going and finding a dog, which gave me something else to distract myself. When we got that little pup that was the best move we made. That was probably the worst I got, just that short period.

Laura didn't say anything at the time, but later on told me that while I was on the hormone treatment I didn't have any affection for her. I didn't really notice that I wasn't paying her any attention. Because of the effects of the drug, it was normal for me. I wasn't interested in sex or having a relationship or cuddling her or anything like that. All interest in Laura was gone; we were just two people walking around the same house. She felt really unloved.

Things didn't turn around until I went off the hormone treatment and we slowly got back to normal. It just took time. Then in 2008, we did a personal development course together to help us with some volunteering work we were doing. It really came out then, to talk about things, not just think about them, and we found our relationship improved so much. It helped us to understand each other better. Each of us does certain things, and we each have positives and negatives. So you just work to focus on the positives and reduce the negatives, and being aware of yourself, what you are thinking and how you are acting.

In this situation you need to talk to each other, that is the main thing, involve your wife, from diagnosis onwards. Every time I go to the doctor's, Laura goes with me, goes into the consultation, and gets all the information as well. If I have to go for scans or anything, Laura goes with me, and she's there and supports me 100% all the way. She was like that from the very beginning.

You need to be patient about sex. Gradually over time after I came off the hormone therapy it came back. I wasn't on the hormone therapy for too long, the longer you are on it, the longer it takes to get back and you have to be really patient. There are other ways to be affectionate though, and you need to look at all that and be aware that you have a partner and they have needs too. And don't blame yourself; it's not your fault.

Laura

As a partner, I am not going through what Jim is going through personally and I don't know exactly what he is going through. I mean, I can see it, but I can't actually feel it. Jim's pretty positive, and because of that I think it does help him a lot. I suppose I try to be happy and try to do things and have a variety of things that we do together — go places not just mope around the house.

I didn't get any support when Jim was diagnosed. We didn't really know what we were doing and we panicked! Now with what we know, I think both of us would have stayed still for a bit, held back and tried to come to terms with it more.

I do think that in a partnership you both need to be really involved. We did notice that a lot of men at medical consultations were there on their own. We would go to the doctors and see men sitting in the waiting room on their own, or sometimes if the wives did come, they would just sit out in the waiting room while the husband went in to see the doctor. I think partners should find out as much as they can about what is going on, because if you don't ask the questions, sometimes the doctor is not going to tell you.

Casey

I was diagnosed with prostate cancer about eighteen months ago, almost by accident. I had experienced a blood clot and so was being put through a number of tests to try and work out why, checking my heart and my blood profile. My heart got the okay and then it was off to the haematologist. My blood tests, a full blood count, came back normal except for a very high PSA result. I was off to the urologist the next day, more tests and a biopsy and then a referral to an oncologist. I started androgen blocking therapy and then had six months of chemotherapy. It was pretty tough going, but I was pragmatic about what had to be done. I never thought about 'Why me?'. It doesn't matter why I have it; I do, so I need to deal with it and get it done.

I am very fortunate to have a supportive partner, and his work was really flexible so that he could come with me to all my appointments and be there when I needed him. I think he took my lead on how we were going to deal with it, but it made a huge difference to me when he said we will be okay and we will get through this together, it was about us, not just me. It is tough on your partner; it is a two-way street. He had to think about what it meant to him to have a partner who has cancer. We made a life commitment to each other, to grow old together, and that's what we still plan to do. My oncologist helped in our attitude by saying to me, 'you are going to live a long and healthy life with a condition' and that's how I think about it.

Sex is important to most men; for gay men we tend to find it easy to talk about sex. We can be flexible in how we approach sex and sexuality, but like in any relationship, there are frustrations and it can be hard. What is harder is finding health professionals who are comfortable talking about gay sex. My partner and I were fortunate in getting early advice and support from a prostate cancer specialist nurse who was amazing — easy going, knowledgeable and supportive. We focus on being close, intimate and if anything, I think our intimacy has increased. We can be close and naked together, an orgasm can be exhilarating and intense, we don't both have to cum, and it can be wonderful.

We cope together and make time to walk by the river, in the warm sunshine and just be together. There are times when I need some space to be by myself, and my partner understands that. Just to recharge and relax in my own way.

One of the hardest things during treatment was the tiredness and fatigue. The treatment itself is taxing and then there are the sleep disruptions because of side effects. It's exhausting. As a result, working was difficult. My Manager and the team I work with were fantastic. I was able to go home early if I was ill or not come in at all. I found it hard during chemo to keep up my exercise routine so just kept walking and keeping active as best I could rather than my gym routine. After chemo I saw an Exercise Physiologist to get a resistance training program and I combine that now with walking. When you are on hormone blockers you have to manage weight gain and muscle loss as well as bone density issues: so prescribed exercise (or exercise medicine) really matters, and a healthy diet. In many ways I am healthier now than I was before my diagnosis. I meditate as well and have found a support group where I can meet men facing the same challenges and share experiences. I do find I cry more easily as a result of the hormone blockers, and I have found from talking to other men from all walks of life that this is a common effect. I think it is important not to label this as a weakness or a problem; it is just the way it is. You need to learn to be comfortable with it. I need to explain to my partner when I am more emotional 'just because of the ADT'.

I think one thing men can do to help themselves is to be informed, and this means being informed about what is relevant to them. I don't think it is helpful to try and compare yourself to others, everyone is different and you can't judge how you are going by comparing PSA test results with other men. I think it is an unhelpful comparison. All cancers are different. But sharing ideas for keeping well physically and emotionally and normalising what you are going through is an enormous benefit.

Chapter 5

How to Make Decisions You can Live With

Imagine you own a sleek red Ferrari. You have owned and loved it for years, driven it a bit too hard and fast at times, neglected it a little of late, and you recently noticed a vague knock in the engine. You take it to a specialist mechanic, a little embarrassed about the state of the duco, but determined to get it fixed and back on the road. The mechanic runs a few tests and says it is actually a pretty serious mechanical problem and he offers you four different options. First, he suggests you could just let it go for a while and see what happens. It might not cause you too much trouble; you could wait and see. Or if you really want to just get it fixed, he has three different approaches that he thinks will all do the job. Each of these three approaches has different possible issues in terms of how long the car will be off the road, the cost, how long the engine will likely go trouble-free, and what might need to be done if the problem recurs. The mechanic gives you a leaflet with all the options and sends you home to think about it.

Sound familiar? It can be a big shock when you are diagnosed with prostate cancer and find out that there are several different treatment options and that you need to be involved in the decision about what treatment to have. This might sound crazy at first. If your car is broken the mechanic usually tells you what needs to be done. That is their job after all. Similarly, you might expect one correct 'fix' to treat a cancer, and you probably expect the doctor to offer you this one best way. Being asked to make this decision yourself is a big call.

One of the first challenges is the medical language that doctors use. Maybe you didn't even really know you had a prostate gland before this, much less exactly where it is (so close to the plumbing) and what it does. The words used to describe cancer and treatments are unfamiliar to most people. Who (other than health professionals) uses words like *carcinoma*, *radical prostatectomy*, and *brachytherapy* in normal day-to-day life? It can be hard to be sure about exactly what the doctor is telling you and what it really means. As well, much of what you will be told is expressed in numbers, percentages or chances of things happening. Even doctors don't always understand these risk estimates, so how hard is it then for a layperson?

Statistics can be misleading and confusing. For example, if you are told that having an extra type of treatment will reduce your chance of the cancer coming back by 50% that sounds pretty worthwhile. But if your chance of the cancer coming back is only 8%, then what the extra drug does is cut that by half to 4%. You might still think this is a path worth taking, but you can see how 50% sounds so much better than 4%. If you read that after surgery the chance of not being able to get an erection is 30%, does that mean you might not get an erection 30% of the time or does it mean three out of ten men won't be able to get an erection? How do you know your chances of being in the 30% anyway?

Aside from being confusing to many, the other thing about percentages and risk numbers is that while they will be the best figures available, they are based on trials and large groups of other people. Not you. So they are an estimate of what might happen, not what will happen. So the uncertainty remains.

Making Decisions under Stress

As a rule, we don't think as clearly when we are stressed, and you don't get much more stress than when you are facing cancer. If you think back to the analogy of a diagnosis of prostate cancer as 'facing a tiger', you are getting ready from a physiological point of view to fight or run. This stress response, as it is often called, is designed to help you keep yourself safe from immediate danger. It is not designed to help you sit down and reflect clearly on all possible actions you might take, weigh up and consider the pros and cons of different approaches, and then choose a carefully laid out plan. Our thinking just does not work as well when we are stressed. If you think of your mind as your workbench — when you are stressed, your 'mental workbench' becomes cluttered. It becomes harder to find things, to make sense of them, and to make a decision. This means that while many men and their partners would prefer a quickly achieved clear plan of action so they can move out of uncertainty and get on with it, this is often not possible.

Ways to Make Decisions

Most of us do not have brains that work like computers — in a programmed, predictive, and logical way. We are much more complicated and interesting than that. The way we make decisions is influenced by our feelings, attitudes, history, what has worked well for us in the past, and how important the decision is.

There are two approaches people tend to apply when making decisions. There is the *systematic* approach, and then there is the *quick shortcut*.

In the systematic approach, we carefully gather information, look at the pros and cons, weigh it all up, and then make a call. Systematic decision making takes effort and time. It can mean a better-informed decision where you are very clear about the choice you made and why. This is the type of decision-making approach often seen as best. An approach where you are well informed about your options, involved in the decision in an equal partnership with your doctor and with the support of the people most close to you. On the other hand, if you have an information overload, it can be easy to get lost and to focus on issues that seem important but actually aren't. As well, taken to the extreme, there is a point where the searching for information can become a type of avoidance — avoiding a decision by looking for certainty or an answer that just isn't there.

If we choose to go for the quick shortcut instead, we usually look for a cue that we might choose to follow. An example would be going for the same option as someone you admire or respect, or who got a good result from their choice. Shortcut decision-making strategies are very useful to have as they are quick and require less effort than the systematic approach. A possible pitfall though is if you use a shortcut and it doesn't work out well, you might later wish you have taken a different approach.

Some people tend to be more systematic; others go more for cues; most of us do a bit of both. How important the decision is and how confident you feel about your ability to make the decision will also influence how you approach the decision.

As an example, when you bought your last car, did you read up on all the latest car reviews, compile a list of all the features that mattered most to you and then match these to each possible car choice? Did you then run a series of test drives and then finally make a choice based on weighing up the pros and cons of each car? If you did, then that was an example of systematic decision making. Or, did you buy a Holden because you are a Holden man and always have been or choose a Toyota because most of your friends drive one and they think they are the most reliable? Both of these last two examples are shortcuts.

So how should I make my decision?

In the best of worlds, you would start by being well informed about your cancer, clear about how much support you need in making the decision from your doctor and your family, and then you would use your support people to help you work this through. A few tips are:

- Take your time. There is seldom a need to make an immediate decision. Talk to your doctor and be clear about your best timeline.
- Be informed. Read up about prostate cancer from reliable sources such as those listed in the Appendix of this book.

- Talk about the decision with your specialist and maybe your GP, and if you are still unclear, go back and ask more questions.
- Feel very comfortable about getting a second opinion if you feel you want an alternative view. You have a right to a second opinion, and most doctors are happy to organise this for you.
- It can be helpful to tape your discussions with your doctor to listen to again at home in case you missed important details.
- Take a support person with you to your doctor's visits. Two heads are better than one!
- Contact a support group and talk to men who have had different treatments so you can get a personal view.
- Be wary of uninformed opinions that can throw you off track.

Activity

Make a list of the treatments your doctor has suggested would be suitable for you. Beside each option list the possible positives (the pros) and the possible negatives (the cons).

Looking at the pros and cons for each, does it look like one option has more pros and fewer cons than the others?

Now put a circle around the pros that matter to you most and the cons that worry you the most. What option looks like it will get you what you value most?

Take this list to your doctor and talk it over with him to make sure you have the facts right. Talk the list over with your partner or someone close to you that you trust. This will help you clarify further what option seems to be closest to your values and will keep your support network in the loop.

Will I regret my decision?

Without a crystal ball, it is not possible to know for sure how you will feel about your decision down the track. However, if you take time and make a carefully considered choice, you will know, whatever happens, that you made the best choice you could in a tough situation.

Personal Stories

Below are personal stories from Geoff and Allan about how they each approached making their decisions about treatment and how they feel about that decision now.

Geoff

I was diagnosed in 2009 and had a radical prostatectomy and dissection of my lymph glands. It was an anxious time, with uncertainty about what the cancer meant for me, and I was also worried about the idea of having surgery. I have had previous problems with deep vein thrombosis, so I was a high risk for surgery in terms of possible complications. So it was a real issue to work out what would be the best treatment for me and how this would affect my partner Barbara. We were both involved in all the consultations, the decision making and all the follow-up. Prayer was very important for both myself and my wife at this time as well.

I read a lot of medical articles, but these articles can't tell you about you as an individual. They are studies about groups of men. What we needed was discussions with the specialists about what the studies meant for us. We saw a total of three doctors — two urologists, they were very different, and I also saw a radiation oncologist. With the second urologist we came away feeling very comfortable with the decision which we discussed at the time and really felt as comfortable as one can with the prospect of surgery. We felt that we had been able to talk and ask questions, and the questions were answered and discussed in a very easy way. It made so much difference for both of us; it really did.

I was well informed and as I said, read up a lot, first about the surgery and the risks involved and how to minimise those. We did a fair bit of work on that and then about the possible side effects of the surgery. It is difficult to get a balance. I think blokes are in two groups — one is men who want surgery and want it removed and out of them. Then the other are men who won't have a bar of surgery and go for the other options. I was worried about incontinence and erectile dysfunction, but it is difficult to actually get a balanced view of all the pros and cons. You know that there are some risks but percentages aren't always easy to understand or helpful. What you can do is find out what the risks are as precisely as you can, through reading and talking to the surgeon, and from this getting a ballpark figure of what you might be facing.

In the end, for me, the big issues were surviving surgery without complications and then facing erectile dysfunction and urinary incontinence. I was at first keen on brachytherapy from the sex point of view, but I thought it would be big trouble because of the urinary difficulty I was having at the time. I chose surgery because I felt surgery would be the only definitive way of knowing the extent of my cancer, and secondly, I was already having urinary problems, difficulty passing water, and I thought that the prostatectomy would get rid of that. I still think this was the best decision for me.

My advice to others is to work on this together, take your time and seek more than one opinion. Be sure you are comfortable with what is happening. Talk to as many people as can, and if you have a support group in your area give it a try. There will be people there who have been through that journey and really have heaps of knowledge and can answer a lot of your questions. Be comfortable with your doctor, and if you are in a relationship, make sure you both know what is going on. This is something that affects you both, and it is really important that you are both in the decision making.

Allan

At the time I was diagnosed with prostate cancer my awareness of the disease was based on the experience of a close friend from my engineering student days. While our lives had taken different paths we were still in contact and I did learn from John in his late 50s that he had undergone a radical prostatectomy and he was getting on with life. 'The disease is easy to diagnose' he advised, 'and you can do something about it if diagnosed with it.'

Just prior to my diagnosis, city-based GP medical centres were starting up and based entirely on the improved flexibility and convenience of securing an appointment, I had decided not to remain with the GP who bought out my retiring GP's practice. The very next time I needed the services of a GP I went to the clinic closest to my office. That occurred on a Saturday morning when consultations were provided without appointment by one of the two doctors rostered on. I was feeling feverish and quite unwell.

I was attended to by a mid-30s female GP. As one component of the consultation, and because I had arrived without any of my medical history, I was asked to undergo a series of tests at a nearby private hospital. One definitive piece of information relevant to this story identified that my PSA was high for my age. While that condition was in no way connected to the medical situation that I was experiencing at the time, it did lead to a visit to a urologist, a DRE and a biopsy. Even though I was entirely without any physical or other symptoms associated with having prostate cancer, its existence was definitively confirmed.

Before my first appointment with the urologist I heard a community announcement over the radio that a prostate cancer support group was to be held that night. I went along. It was the first of many steps on the journey that I took to become as informed as possible about prostate cancer, treatment options, implications of side effects of treatment, treatment impacts on my employment, emotional highs and lows, survivor stories and survival statistics.

When my prostate cancer was confirmed I was already conditioned to accept that possibility purely on the statistical chance when considered within the context of my sex and age range. I was 65 years of age. Gaining an understanding that the cancer's characteristics did have a logical structure was an engaging experience. Most of its descriptors are defined either numerically or in relative terms — the PSA, the Gleason Score, the Stage of the disease, the volume of the prostate, the number of biopsy cores that were positive, and the urine flow. That awareness was comforting because we engineers work well with stats and I found that my predicament could be somewhat demystified!

Treatment options in my community were relatively limited at that time — essentially open surgery, radiation or hormone therapy. I was advised by the urologist that for my particular circumstances, I would be a good candidate for either surgery or radiation. My overall health and fitness were good and there were no physical or emotional situations that might have complicated the choice of treatment. The prediction was that I could expect very similar outcomes from either of the two available treatments of surgery and external beam radiation therapy. Through the above interaction with the urologist I gained a reasonable understanding of how the surgery option would impact on my daily living, my post-treatment recovery and my return to work.

At that time, I was working on an assignment that required intermittent on-site involvement in a regional country area. I obtained a comparable consultation from a radiation oncologist and formed the view that the radiation option offered scope for lifestyle considerations appropriate to my circumstances that the surgery option precluded. Radiation did not require me to cease working for any treatment at any time. If I took this option I could continue my pattern of early gym workouts three mornings a week. I could also vary the timing of treatment sessions to suit my schedule.

Accordingly, the decision to choose radiation for my treatment was made on lifestyle factors that were important to my family and me at the time. To me, prostate cancer was not immediately life-threatening. The impact was decidedly more life confronting. Just what was I being required to deal with? Where would I get the information and support that I would require? Who were the specialists that I would consult with — the professionals, and those with lived experiences?

I was being required to make a call on what I understood, not the whole spectrum of what was involved. In life, engineers can be required to make important decisions on a daily basis. They work within the context of a whole range of competencies provided by others on whom we routinely rely — designers, manufacturers and operators. So what is so different in terms of the process of deciding on your choice of treatment for your prostate cancer?

I took three months to decide on my choice of treatment. I took advice from health care professionals, I listened to the experiences of men who had travelled the journey before me, and I took account of lifestyle choices that were important to my family and me. No medical practitioner could have made that decision for me. I did not deliberate at length on possible side effects of treatment that might be experienced down the track. I felt the downsides of worrying about what you just don't know could have a greater negative impact on me than the disease itself.

I made the decision that determined the start of my prostate cancer journey of treatment and survival success. At the same time, I made a commitment to prepare myself to deal with issues not yet defined, as and when it became important for me to do so, and that would involve ongoing inclusion of health care specialists, desk research and learning from others who were still travelling a journey that I had yet to experience.

Chapter 6

Sex: 'What now?'

Sex is important. Without reproduction we would eventually cease to exist. The survival of the human race depends on sex. This means that biologically as adults, we are all at some level sexual beings, even if we are not in a sexual relationship and regardless of our sexual orientation. As thinking beings though (with large brains) there is for all of us a more complicated social and relational side to sex.

We are bombarded much of the time with messages about sex. If we go to the movies or watch television, there is a good chance we will see a warning about nudity and sexual references, which most of us don't even always notice. We have advertisements on billboards and television and in magazines from people trying to sell us things by inferring that there is a link between sex and their product. The messages include: 'If we wear this deodorant, drive this car or motorbike, or even if we live in a certain type of apartment, then we will be sexier and more successful in love. While we kind of know these ads aren't really true, who has never succumbed wishfully and given it a go?

These days it's pretty hard to get away from sex, or the idea of sex, no matter what our background or views are around this sensitive topic. Sex is ubiquitous.

However, despite all this exposure (and how important sex is for the species) for many of us, sex is not an easy topic to talk about. This is somewhat ironic given how much time in our lives we spend thinking about it, avoiding it, worrying about it, looking for it, or enjoying it! As we grow up, we learn a lot of rules about sex (often unspoken but clear nonetheless) from our parents and our peers. This includes rules about what sort of sex is okay, when it is okay and with whom, and how we should think or talk about sex. These rules have a big influence on how we manage sex in our lives, and they are not always helpful to us. This may be even more so when sex and making love becomes difficult or more complicated because of cancer treatments or because our bodies are ageing and have started to work a little differently. When this happens, we need to learn new ways of having sex. However, communicating and experimenting do not often come naturally.

How Sex Might Change

Feeling ourselves to be sexual beings is often a central part of who we are, our identity, and for many is associated with a sense of youth and vitality. Changes to the sexual part of ourselves can lead to a huge sense of loss, and working this through can be tough. You might already be struggling with this just because of ageing and the physiological and physical appearance changes that occur for both men and women. Let's go over these briefly.

Although men get more leeway to look 'distinguished' as they become older, gravity hits everyone, and men may get more fat around the middle and lose some muscle — the usual list for all but the super fit. Testosterone also declines with age, especially in men who are not physically fit. Sexual desire is often not as strong and the amount of ejaculate is less. It can take longer to get an erection and your erection may not be as strong or as persistent. Orgasms can at times seem less intense. In men, the ability to get and keep hard erections is closely tied to cardiovascular (blood vessel) health. Men who have high blood pressure, diabetes, clogged arteries, a lot of belly fat, and who smoke or drink too much alcohol are much more likely to get erection problems with ageing.

All of this is going on at just the age when prostate cancer is most likely to hit. And then we discover that perhaps the most pronounced negative physical effect of prostate cancer treatments is on sex.

For women, decreases in the female sex hormones as they go through menopause can make sex less pleasurable. Vaginal lubrication often decreases, and the lining of the vagina thins and is less elastic, making penetration tight or painful.

Sexual desire or libido may also decrease, although life stress may be more important than hormones in women's interest and energy for sex. If you are not in the mood or sex is painful, it can be harder to reach an orgasm.

As well as this, let's be honest, we live in a culture that celebrates youth as beauty and idealises younger women. In these times, as an older woman, you can feel a bit invisible. As we age our whole body changes in other ways, and it's not just our hormones. Gravity hits, fat starts to appear in unhelpful places, and we start to lose muscle tone and strength. It is hard to feel interested in sex and romance if you feel sexually unattractive or uninteresting and not valued in this way.

How Prostate Cancer affects Sex

The prostate gland sits snugly around the base of the bladder and so is right in the middle of the nerves and blood supply needed for an erection. This means that surgery and radiation therapy for prostate cancer can have a direct effect on a man's ability to get or maintain an erection. There are plenty of easy to find booklets and web pages that outline exactly how and why this happens, but this is the nub of it. A man might find after treatment that he is unable to get or keep a hard erection or that his erections are unreliable. This can be devastating. If a man has radiation therapy for a time, orgasms might be painful, and the rectal area may be painful or irritated. For all men who have had treatment, the amount of ejaculate will lessen and after surgery to remove the prostate ejaculations will be dry.

If a man is on hormone-blocking treatment, he will find his desire for sex reduces as well as his erections, making it even more difficult to keep an active, pleasurable sex life.

It is important to be clear about this: these are physical treatment effects. They are not 'in your head'. To solve them, you will probably need to use medical treatments. There are a range of pills, medicines that can be injected into the penis, sexual aids like vacuum pumps, and even surgery to put a penile implant (pump system) inside a man's body. The main point is that this is something that will require medical help. As well, most doctors now advise that getting the blood flow back to the penis early in recovery is important for long term erectile function. Therefore, thinking about this sooner rather than later is a good idea.

There is a psychological side as well, though. The worry of a cancer diagnosis itself can reduce sexual interest, just as you might have found when other tough things have happened in your life. Many men report feeling that if they can't get an erection, they are not sexually interesting or capable and that this stops them from even thinking sexy thoughts.

Finally, sex after prostate cancer needs more planning, understanding, and communication within a couple, as well as medical help. If lovemaking doesn't work so well in the early days, some couples find they feel less inclined to persist in trying and just give up.

Why bother?

This is really up to you. Some couples do say that they had become less interested in sex before the cancer anyway and that they have talked it over now and decided it was time to give away having sex. For these couples, physical closeness, affection and comfort stay an important part of their lives, with cuddling, kissing, and lots of hugs becoming their main way of keeping physically close and connected.

For other couples, keeping an active sex life matters. If you want to stay sexually active, or you can see that your partner is frustrated about sex, there is a lot you can do. The key things are to talk about it, be informed, be patient with each other, flexible in your approach and open to new things — and to start early. The sooner you get to work on this, the more likely you will be to succeed.

How do I get started?

When all this is going on it is easy for a couple to have misunderstandings about sex. A man who is worried about whether he can perform sexually might become withdrawn and stop initiating sex. His partner, however, might see this as rejection and feel hurt and frustrated. Talking honestly with each other about how sex and love-making have changed and how you would each like sex to be is the first step.

The next step is to be informed about the physical effects of prostate cancer treatments and what treatments and aids are available to help you with these effects. Some useful resources are listed in the Appendix in this book. Your doctor will have advice and be able to guide you about what treatments might work best for you and may also refer you to a doctor who specialises in sexual health.

Sex is a mutual activity, so if you are in a relationship you need to work on this as a couple. This means at the outset talking with each other about the options you have and working out which might suit you both best. In the previous chapter, I talked about ways to make informed decisions about treatment, and these strategies can be applied here as well. In brief, this means be clear about and list your options, work out the pros and cons, weigh up what you think suits you both best, work closely with your doctor on the plan and be ready to change the plan as needed. Too many men try a treatment for a sexual problem but give up when it does not restore them right away to their memories of being age twenty. You and your partner may need to try several different treatments before you find one that satisfies you both.

This does not mean though that you should turn having sex into work. When you do put the plan in place, make sure to also do the fun romantic things to add a little zing. It does not have to mean a second honeymoon. Just putting a high priority on time for talking, maybe a nice dinner, dancing in the dark to romantic music, fun in a hot tub, watching a sexy movie, and above all, plenty of time and privacy.

Be aware that being anxious about having sex after prostate cancer is normal but may not be helpful. Taking time to keep physical closeness a part of your life without feeling pressured about sexual performance is crucial. Remember that sex does not have to include penetration, and sex roles may need to change. Many couples find other ways to give each other sexual pleasure that is both satisfying and helps them keep a feeling of being physically close and intimate. This is what this chapter's Activity is about.

What if I don't have a partner?

If you don't currently have a partner this does not mean that you will never have one again. So if this is your situation, it is still important for you to understand how treatment has affected your erectile function and libido and what you can do about this. You may be concerned that you are now less attractive as a sexual partner and be fearful of rejection. And it can be tricky working out when to broach the subject with a new partner and talk about how sex works for you now. As well, it can be hard just letting someone new know you have had cancer, let alone talking about sexual changes. There are no easy answers to this except to say that preparation will help, so practising how you might raise the topic and discuss it is a good idea. Many men have told me that although they were nervous about starting a new relationship, with the right person and good communication, they have been able to connect and have satisfying sex and intimate friendships.

Activity

Set aside time to talk about how you are each feeling about your sexual lives and how you would like things to be in the best of worlds. This is best not done in the bedroom, where you might each feel a little tense. Try talking about this over a cup of coffee or a relaxing drink after dinner. You need privacy and to pick a time when you won't be interrupted. The goal here is to agree on what steps you would like to take as a couple to get sex back on track. Once you agree, you can start to make a plan about what external medical help you would like, get informed about the options, and try out options that suit you both. Think of your options as a menu (perhaps French!) to choose from. Be prepared to try different approaches until you find one that you are both happy with.

When you are trying to get back to a normal sex life, it helps to start by making time to give each other physical, sensual pleasure without having actual sex. For this activity sexual touch is banned! Set aside at least one hour for private physical touch time. You need a private place like your bedroom, there needs to be no interruptions, and you both need to agree that the next hour (or two) is for giving and receiving pleasure through physical touch. Candles, soft mood lighting and relaxing music are a good start as well as a state of undress to the extent you are comfortable. Now take turns touching and massaging your partner in non-sexual places, fifteen to twenty minute turns each. Notice how good it feels to touch and be touched, and to give and receive pleasure. Talk to each other (compliments are good) and have fun with this. This exercise is about being close and feeling good about yourself and each other.

When you are comfortable with touching in places that are less 'sexual', try different ways of giving and receiving sensual pleasure short of having actual sexual intercourse. This can include touching each other on sensitive and sexual parts of the body and giving pleasure through physical stimulation using hands or your mouth. Be playful. Instead of worrying about reaching an orgasm, just focus on learning new ways to give each other pleasure. Ask each other what feels good and work on learning what kinds of touch your partner prefers. For this exercise, sexual intercourse is not the goal. The goal is finding ways to give sexual or sensual pleasure to each other that do not rely on having an erection or achieving penetration. It is about intimacy and trust.

Personal Stories

Following are personal stories from Barbara and Geoff about how they approached getting their sex life back on track after treatment. Brad shares his experience as a young gay man diagnosed with prostate cancer and how he needed to rewire his thinking. Finally, a story with a touch of humour in it from Ian, whose main message is get on to it early!

Barbara

Geoff had a radical prostatectomy in 2009, and my feelings at the time focussed on getting rid of the cancer. My concerns were for Geoff at the actual time of the surgery and for his health during the operation, but also what was going to happen afterwards and how were we going to cope.

Our sex life was great; it was really exciting and really good. The idea of how that was going to work after surgery I suppose wasn't initially worrying me, but afterwards was more on my mind. We didn't address this until well after surgery; we just thought we could do something about it if we found Geoff couldn't get an erection afterwards. I heard a lot about the various things you can do, but we didn't go into the detail. It didn't seem relevant, and we thought we would just have to tackle that when we came to it.

We were able to get a lot of comprehensive information about couple and sexuality issues from a couples support trial we were in, and that helped us enormously. We worked through the information independently and then talked about it as a couple. The way it was presented and authored was terrific. We also had the opportunity to speak together for perhaps an hour at a time and share the issues that were concerning us with a mentor that was so important. I think it made a lot of difference to our openness with one another.

The mentor also gave us practical tips, like talking more, taking out time for us as a couple. Our lives were busy and still are busy. But making a special time in our week, in our day, to talk about our sex life, things we can try, how did it work for each one of us, what was good, what was not so good, really helped. Listening more to one another as well, that also made a huge difference. These are very practical ideas, things that we thought we were doing pretty well, to be honest — but having a mentor and having someone else to share with made us realise that there was more we could do.

Support groups can help as well. I know in our own support group people are very open in talking about sexual issues and the problems that they are facing.

I think openness and genuineness, being genuine with each other is really, really important. You can't afford to hold back. I think you have to be quite open about sex and I can understand how people could find that very difficult. For me, this is essential as part of being a couple, having a partner, and having someone to share your life with.

Geoff

We have always been very open in talking about sex and everything else as far as that goes. When we went back to the surgeon for the six-week check-up we started to ask what we could be doing to help matters along. Indeed at that stage, we saw a colleague of my urologist who took us for an hour to talk about what we might be able to do.

I think as a first step you have to talk about it with each other. You've got to be prepared; I mean it can't come as a great shock or surprise. You have to think through what you want as a couple before you embark and discuss it with the doctor.

One practical thing that I think is very relevant is to see a specialist about it. We saw a surgeon who suggested I see a colleague of his who specialised in erectile problems. We spent a long time with that fellow talking about what we could do about it, right from the start, right after the post-operative visit. It was very helpful.

I agree with Barbara that the support trial reinforced everything that we thought we had been doing. It refocused us at a time when we had tried some things about erectile dysfunction and things hadn't been going too well. It brought us back to address the issue and actually made us make some progress. The mentor also gave us some very practical tips which helped us to make progress on the matter. We could have dropped it at that stage and said, 'oh well, you know that's it for sex'. But we persevered through that and got some support to give us the means and strategies to solve the sexual problems we faced. Rather than thinking we've hit a dead-end, we thought there were some other avenues to explore. We also got some very good tips from the counsellor about the penile injections and the vacuum pump.

It was really worth the effort and focus, and now we are very happy with how things are going in this area of our lives. But we do have to stay focussed and we don't take it for granted.

Brad

I was only 46 years old when I was diagnosed, and as a young gay man I think the hardest thing was the sense of isolation. It seemed to me that everything I read about prostate cancer was aimed at heterosexual older men, and so I was an outlier, or so I thought at the time. My GP had been testing me regularly since I was 40 years old, and he detected that I had an enlarged prostate and a rising PSA. I had a biopsy, and cancer was found. It was really hard to get my head around it. I was single and so had no partner to support me. I did however have a very close friend, and my father was also very supportive. They helped me get through it all. The treatment I chose was radical prostatectomy, and I did pretty well I think. My incontinence settled after about three to four weeks, and within five weeks I got my potency back as well although it's not the same as before. Once you lose your prostate you can still orgasm, but you don't ejaculate, and this is a loss. Your sex life changes in other ways as well and might need some discussion with prospective partners. But you get there, and the right guys don't worry. With sex, it is the way you think about it that can cause you the most trouble rather than the reality.

I felt embarrassed and ashamed for some time and very anxious. As a gay man, you face a lot and already can feel invisible. You can get sensitised to shame. After my diagnosis it was like my masculinity or sense of myself as a man was shaken, that I was inadequate. At first I tried to keep it a secret. I saw a psychologist for some time to help me work this through. I was ruminating and worrying, thinking I will never have a partner or have sex again, catastrophising that the cancer would be the end of me, that I wouldn't survive it. Ten years later, I can tell you none of this was actually true. I had to challenge these negative thoughts and reframe how I looked at myself and my experience. I had to rewire my thinking. I also took steps to look after myself better and build my general resilience. I cut down on alcohol, reached out to my friends and family for support, and I got involved in a support group. Helping others helped me.

It is not helpful when people tell you to just get over it. It takes time. The issues are more than just survival, your quality of life matters. Facing this and working this through is difficult. I learnt that I was stronger than I thought and that I had the courage to face this. As a young man with prostate cancer, I found my voice.

My advice to other men is to be informed, read up from reliable sources, and get good medical advice. Information is power. Look after yourself with exercise and healthy eating. Lean on the people around you who care about you. Reach out for support.

Like me, you can find your courage and your voice. You are not alone, and you are more than you might think.

Ian

I underwent a robotic prostatectomy in May 2009. I went through the usual urinary leakage (more like a flood at times) which gradually decreased. After six months, I began to feel like having sex again, however I could not get much of an erection and certainly could not maintain it for long when I did manage to have a partial one. I tried Viagra and other pills, and a vacuum pump which didn't help. I looked at penile injections but decided I didn't want to go sticking those in my penis (it had had enough I thought).

As time went on with no improvement I became very angry and morose. I had been through all this just to face impotency. My relationship with my wife deteriorated and my work suffered. Approximately nine months after the operation, I went to see my urologist for a check-up and asked him about an implanted pump. His reaction was that there was no need. All I really needed were the injections and that they weren't the issue I had built them up to be. He gave me a referral to a men's health doctor. I think I made the appointment as I was walking out his door.

My first encounter with this men's health doctor was a revelation and a riot. He spent some time explaining the process in detail and then he showed me how to inject myself. We started with a dosage just under the maximum. There it was — a thing of beauty and a joy forever (well, the forever part was right). After I had gloried in the sensation for some time, he convinced me that I should inject the antidote. I then left his office (both hands in my pockets) and went back to my own office. The doctor had given me tablets to take if the erection did not go away. It didn't, so I took the tablets and then remembered that I had a meeting scheduled with two women. It was too late to cancel!

With a strategically placed manila folder, I entered the meeting room, quickly sat down and made sure that my errant and rampant erection was securely out of sight under the table. At the end of the meeting (still rampant) I then had to juggle shaking hands, saying goodbye and the manila folder. I then made a beeline to my office and phoned the doctor. I returned to his office (both hands in my pockets) and he gave me another injection of antidote.

After that I experimented with lower and lower dosage levels until I had worked out what was the best for a comfortable erection that went away after a reasonable time. My sex life and my attitude improved exponentially. Over three years from the original operation, I still use small doses of the serum for a fantastic result. If I had had the courage to bring the subject up directly with my urologist and started the injections earlier, I would not have gone through so much mental turmoil and my life would have returned to normal much more quickly. My advice, don't put it off!

Chapter 7

'I think therefore I am!'

(cogito ergo sum[1]*)*

When Rene Descartes wrote these very famous words in 1644 the key point was — if I can think, I must exist. That this phrase gets used so very often in so many different situations speaks to how important the act of thinking is to who we are and how we exist in the world.

So thinking is important, but further to this *how* we think is important and influences how we feel and act in response to what goes on around us.

Imagine this scenario:

> You wake up and get ready for work, go down to the car driveway and the car is not there! Someone must have stolen it! You start to panic, you keep the fuel card in the car, and whoever has the car can go anywhere. Your whole week will be ruined; you had a weekend planned away with your partner, and a big meeting at work this morning that you will be late for. Your boss will be furious. You can feel your heart

[1] Originally written in French, but later translated into Latin, the philosophical statement was described by Descartes as meaning: "We cannot doubt of our existence while we doubt;" the idea being that if you can doubt your existence and are able to think about this you must therefore exist.

> racing, and you feel sick in the stomach. Why do bad things always happen to me? You run inside to call the police and then your partner reminds you that you caught the bus home yesterday and left the car at work.

How often have you hit the panic button only to find your worse fear was not true or did not happen?

Most of the time we think in an automatic way, without effort, and in patterns we have learned and practised all our lives. How many times have you reflected that someone you know (or maybe even you) always thinks the worst, or the best, or jumps to conclusions? It matters because we do tend to respond as if our thoughts are absolutely true, and if our mind perceives a tiger out there, our bodies will react as if there really is one and will set off the physical stress response accordingly. You can test this out for yourself in the following simple thinking exercise.

Activity

> First, think about something that happened in the past that was really upsetting. Remind yourself where this was, who was there and think about what happened and what was said. Think and remember what happened. How do you feel right now after thinking about this?
>
> Now think about something that you would really like to happen, something you have dreamed about. Who would be there with you, and where would you be? What feelings do these thoughts and images bring up in you at this moment?

For both of these exercises, the reality of who and where you are right now didn't change, but how you feel probably did. The only thing that did change was what you were thinking about. How we think and what we think about affects how we feel.

Thinking Patterns

We learn as we grow up how to think and be in the world. If the main message we received was that the world is not a safe place, or that we are not worthwhile, then the way we think and react may be to be hyper-vigilant for danger or to tend to blame ourselves or feel guilty when things go wrong.

On the other hand, if we were mostly led to believe that by and large things will be okay in the long run and that we are competent and able to surmount most things, we might be less likely to jump to the worst possible conclusions.

However you think or react to situations; this is not about saying one way is better or worse. However, if you predict or assume the worse most or much of the time, this is not only upsetting but also exhausting!

There are some common thinking patterns people use that just don't help when you are in a stressful situation.

- ***Catastrophising.*** Thinking of the worst possible outcome that could happen
- ***Black and White Thinking*** (also called 'all or nothing thinking' or 'my way or the highway'). Thinking that things have to go a certain way or it will be a complete disaster.
- ***Self-blame.*** Think that it is all your fault

- *Overgeneralising*. Taking one event and turning it into a sweeping generalisation about how things will always be
- *The Negative Mental Filter*. Seeing only the negative aspects of a situation and ignoring all of the positives
- *Jumping to Conclusions*. Assuming something is negative when there is actually not much evidence to support it.

The trouble with these patterns of thinking is that they can lead you to feel anxious or depressed and that they don't lead you to generate other possibilities or help you look at things in a balanced way. They are pretty much 'dead-end' thinking. And they can also keep you awake late at night when all is quiet and there is nothing to distract you from thinking the worst.

A Different Approach

A different approach is to pick up the habit of checking your thinking for distortion. (Now don't go overboard on this, there is such a thing as too much introspection!) When you notice yourself feeling down or on edge or angry, ask yourself — 'What am I thinking about to make me feel this way?' Secondly, ask yourself — 'Is my way of thinking about my current situation helping me or hindering me? Is this a typical way that I react to situations?' This is the first step. Then, if you do identify unhelpful thoughts that are recurring or causing you to worry more, then challenge them. Say to yourself — 'How true is this thought really, and how helpful is this thought to me? Is there a better way for me to think about this? What would my best friend, or someone I really respect, say to me if they could read my thoughts?'

A good example of the above approach would be if you find yourself thinking something along the lines of, 'I am not going to initiate sex with my partner because it won't work and then they will think I am worthless as a mate'. This is a combination of catastrophising and all-or-nothing thinking. Another example is recollecting all of the times that your partner seemed tired or got cross with you over the week and thinking 'They are not coping and it is all my fault'. This is a combination of using a negative mental filter and jumping to conclusions.

You could start to challenge this thinking by reminding yourself of all the things about each other that you both value outside of sex, such as companionship and family ties. You could also remember that you know sex after prostate cancer takes time and patience and effort and that this is not your fault or anyone else's. (Get the idea?)

Thinking as Processing

However, all of this does not mean you should never have a negative thought. This would be ridiculous. Negative thoughts about your cancer can't physically hurt you, they are just thoughts, and they don't make your cancer worse, just in case anyone has thrown that old chestnut at you. There is no evidence to support the idea that negative thoughts about cancer make the cancer worse.

It is normal for people to, at times, have what we call 'intrusive thoughts' about their cancer. These are unwanted negative thoughts about the cancer that just pop into your head often when you least expect it. These thoughts are most likely just normal mental processing of what is for anyone a 'big deal' life issue. In other words, this is a normal and necessary part of coming to terms with cancer and accepting this as now part of your life history. Trying desperately to never think a negative thought or to even think at all about the cancer (this is given the fancy name of 'cognitive or thought avoidance') increases the likelihood that that thought will continue to pop up and cause even more distress.

Intrusive negative thoughts are really only a problem if they are driving ongoing strong feelings of distress, or are getting in the way of you having a happy life. It doesn't help you if the minute you get a negative thought about the cancer you beat yourself up about it. Remember, they are just thoughts.

Another approach with negative thoughts is to notice they are there, perhaps even label the thought —'Ah Ah! There I go again, thinking that it is all my fault that my partner is tired' and then deliberately shift your focus elsewhere to where you are right now in this very moment. In brief, leave the past and the future to worry about themselves. Live for the now and in the present moment — stop to smell the roses.

Activity

For the next week, keep notes in your journal of the times when you find yourself feeling more upset or stressed. Jot down the day and time, where you are and who you are with, what is going on and most importantly, what you are thinking and feeling.

After a week of keeping these notes, take some time to look them over and see if you can identify a pattern. Do you have a typical way of thinking that you can identify? Are there any of the negative common thinking patterns mentioned above? Are your thoughts realistic or based on accurate or true and known information? Are these thoughts helping or hindering you? Is there a way you could think about what is happening that would serve you better?

Talk this over if you can with your partner or a close and trusted friend. Ask them to support you in coming up with a more helpful view of what is going on. If you don't feel you can talk about these thoughts with someone else, or just prefer not to, become your own best friend. Write down a different way to look at the problem or challenge you are facing that expresses kindness and care to yourself.

Now, find some time in the next week to sit in the garden or go for a short walk. As you do this, notice what is around you. Focus your attention on the finer details of the trees or plants, how the wind plays with your surroundings, and how the sunlight falls and changes the colours around you. Are there small animals you notice, ants or lizards? What noises can you hear? Is there traffic in the distance? Can you hear laughter in the background and the sounds of your own breathing? Now notice how you feel. Practice using this grounding technique next time that you notice getting carried away with negative thoughts.

Personal Stories

Following is a personal story from a different David about his prostate cancer experience and how he has learnt to manage worrying thoughts and keep stress under control.

David

I was diagnosed in 1999 and had a radical prostatectomy in 2000. It was a pretty tough time, and while I had a great surgeon technically, his communication skills could have been better! I had the idea that I had to have the surgery as quickly as possible or the cancer would kill me, and my 'headspace' was exploding! I know now that that wasn't actually the case, I wasn't on death's door, and I could have taken my time a little more.

The main problems I had after surgery were urinary continence and impotence. At the time the urinary continence was my biggest concern. Back then, I wasn't in touch with a support group, and so this meant I had to search out information for myself, with not much help to be honest. I looked on the internet, read books, and then got myself to a physiotherapist to learn pelvic floor exercises, and over time, about twelve months, the problem resolved. My GP was a help as well.

A challenge here was managing my thinking. I have always had a tendency to worry. My mother was like this and I think I learnt this way of thinking from her. I guess I am a natural worrier! All those 'what ifs?' scare the hell out of you. 'What if I never get my urine control back and I have to wear pads for the rest of my life? What if people I know see me buying incontinence pads? What if it gets worse? What if I leak in public?' You can really get into a dark place psychologically if you let these types of thoughts take over.

The way I have taught myself to manage this is first to notice and be more aware of my thinking patterns. None of this comes naturally to me. I have had to learn to do this. Even after all these years, I still do keep an eye on myself for this because worries about the cancer do come back from time to time. When I notice I am doing negative 'what if' type of thinking, I tell myself to stop it and either distract myself by reading a good thriller (great for distraction!) or do something physical like wash the car or walk the dog. Sometimes I just change the subject in my head or change the thought by rationalising. I tell myself that the worrying thought just isn't true and I try and talk to myself in a more positive way. I kind of remind myself that none of this is the end of the world, hard things happen in life and that is just the way of it. I guess I now see having had prostate cancer in that way — as a phase of life I have been through. I do believe that you are in charge of your own destiny. There is no good fairy flitting around to fix things for you. If you want it fixed you need to do it yourself.

I moved cities after my cancer. Having cancer made me reassess how I was living and I decided I wanted less stress and a better quality of life. Cancer made me really realise I was not going to live forever and it was like a little light switched on in my head. My priorities changed, and work didn't seem like the main game anymore. It was a good move for me.

I have always been pretty curious about life and open to what it has to teach me. I am pretty lucky to have a great family, good friends, and I make sure that I keep connected to them; that helps as well. My friends and family are my anchors. When I retired, that was tough as well. I was bored and cranky, irritable and angry a fair bit of the time — not much fun to be around. I worked it out though, did some part-time work for a while and tried different things. It was a big transition. I volunteer now and run a prostate cancer support group, and I feel like this is a really worthwhile thing to do. It is still hard for many men to find support when they need it. Our group helps them see that prostate cancer is not the end of everything. Blokes often come to our group pretty downcast, but after seeing other men doing well, they feel reassured, and becoming better informed makes the lights really go on!

Chapter 8

De-Stressing: How to Look After Yourself and Keep Well

It is probably fair to say that many of us spend a lot of time and energy working, looking after family, getting jobs done, keeping house, and not much time (or enough time) taking care of our health. How many times have you either told yourself, or been advised by others, that you need to relax more, take time out to de-stress, exercise more regularly, and eat better? It is easy to brush this off as a nice idea but one that will need to wait until later — when things settle down, are less busy and you can finally find that time for yourself.

I suspect most of us think this way. The problem however is that this is a delaying tactic. You might never get around to the task of looking after yourself in this way, and so you just keep on 'keeping on' and getting a little more tired, tense, and less at your best as time goes on. The time to look after your health will never be right unless you claim it and make it so. So do it now!

Why bother? Because letting physical and mental tension build-up without a break is like driving your car or motorbike at full throttle all day, every day, no matter what the circumstances. The outcome of this (at least in a motor vehicle) is that the engine wears quickly, the brakes will soon lose their effectiveness, you go through too much petrol, and eventually, the thing just stops, or even worse you lose control. You would not treat your car this way, so why do this to your body?

Looking after your physical and mental wellbeing is important for everyone, but especially important if you are going through the stressful experience of either being diagnosed with cancer or supporting someone who has cancer.

The first aim then in looking after yourself is to reduce *physical tension* in your body. Think back to the earlier chapter in this book that overviewed the stress response. When you are under pressure and in a situation of threat, your body reacts by pumping itself up with action hormones (the 'flight or fight' response) that create physical tension. Not only is this unpleasant to experience, if it goes on unchecked, it is also not good for your overall health. So there is a very good pragmatic reason to use strategies or tools to reduce unwanted or unnecessary physical body tension.

The second aim, and this is just as important, is to reduce *mental tension* and try to clear your mind of worrying thoughts at least some of the time. Mental tension can drive or increase physical tension in a reinforcing cycle, so you need to target both aspects.

There are lots of ways to relax — if you Google relaxation techniques (the last time I checked) you will get 190 million hits! You will have your own usual ways of relaxing, and this might include reading, watching movies, playing golf or bowls, dancing or socialising. If you have let these activities slip in the 'busy-ness' of coping with the cancer, or life in general, then now is a good time to get back on track. Make time in your schedule to do the things that you enjoy and find relaxing. As well though, you might consider learning some new skills or taking on some new activities that are specifically about reducing tension and looking after your physical and mental well-being.

Learning to Relax — Practice makes Perfect

With all dedicated relaxation techniques, it is a good idea to practice them first in a private and quiet place where you won't get disturbed, and in comfortable clothes. As well, don't wait until you are stressed and tense to give it a go. Try it out when you already feel pretty calm until you get the hang of it. Learning relaxation techniques is in some ways like learning to ride a bicycle for the first time — it feels strange. And you are not sure if you are getting it right until suddenly you get an 'Ah-Ha' moment — your body and mind put it all together, and it starts to feel like second nature. So keep the trainer wheels on for a while and practice regularly while you learn how to control your body and mind in this way. Once you get more experienced and skilful you will find that you are able to more effortlessly apply these strategies when you need them the most.

Take a Breath

Controlling and slowing your breath is a very simple way to calm your body. Breathing techniques are easy to do anywhere and anytime, and because they are not obvious to those around you, they can be done in almost any situation of stress and you won't look weird!

As a first step, find a comfortable and quiet place to sit and focus for a few minutes on being aware of your breathing. Notice how the breath moves in and out of your nose and chest, and how your chest muscles contract and relax as you breathe. Listen to the sound of your breath as you breathe in and out. Be aware of your posture and how your shoulders sit as you breathe. If your shoulders are tight and hunched drop them down on your out-breath.

Next, count slowly to four in every *in* and *out*-breath you take. Focus your mind on the count, and breathe in a slow and relaxed and comfortable way in time to the count. Do this for several minutes as your body gets used to slow and controlled breathing.

Now stop and notice how you feel. This is a quick and easy de-stress strategy that can be easily applied to good effect when stuck in traffic, waiting in a doctor's office for a check-up, or at night just before you go to sleep to relax yourself down.

This exercise can be extended by adding in at the end, for a few breaths only, holding your breath for a count of two. You can also add visualisation or imagery by focusing your mind on a safe and relaxing scenario or image towards the end of the exercise, once your breathing has slowed down. This might mean building a picture in your mind of a relaxing place and activity, such as swimming in the sea or walking in a forest, and imagining the colours and sounds and physical sensations you would experience if you were there.

There are of course other techniques you might try, such as progressive relaxation. This approach is where you progressively tense and relax different areas of your body, often starting at the toes and working your way up. The best thing about breathing exercises, and why I tend to teach these first, is that in my experience most people can get the hang of it and get a good effect pretty quickly. If you would like to really broaden your skills in this though you might also want to try meditation techniques.

Meditation and Mindfulness

Meditation originated thousands of years ago and can be described as an approach to life and people that encompasses acceptance, self-knowledge and awareness, love free from expectation, 'letting go' or non-attachment, and at a higher level the search for enlightenment.

Meditation techniques are the central tool in the Buddhist toolbox for life, and these focus on calming the mind. The purpose, generally speaking, is to gain a deeper sense of awareness of the self and the world through stilling the mind. This leads to improved wellbeing and greater resilience to challenges and the problems life can throw at you.

More recently some of these ideas have been packaged as 'mindfulness' where the focus is deliberately paying attention to the present moment, or moment-by-moment awareness without judgement, in a way that leads to a better ability to manage thoughts and feelings.

It might sound a little vague, but there is good evidence that mindfulness and related meditation approaches can improve wellbeing, so it is well worth considering and trying out. As with all relaxation techniques it does tend to be 'horses for courses'. What suits one person may not suit another — it is a very individual thing. However, being open to these ideas and what they might bring for you is another good way of being your own best friend.

Try this quick mindfulness exercise and see how you go!

Activity

Find a place in the garden or a quiet room where you can sit comfortably and uninterrupted for about ten minutes. The goal of this exercise is to stop and become aware of your physical location and your surroundings sense-by-sense. Before you start, check your watch.

First, become aware of how you feel now that you have stopped what you were doing. What thoughts — or echoes of thoughts — have you carried with you into this moment and what feelings are here now? Perhaps scan your body and notice if there are any points of tightness or tension in your body. Next — deliberately gather your attention and redirect it to the feeling of your breath as it enters, and then again, as it leaves your body. Do this for several breaths — almost as if you are dropping anchor into this moment using your breath. Now expand your awareness around your breath and begin to notice how you feel physically in this space. Are you cool or warm? Feel the bottom of your feet and how your feet feel against the ground. Are you sitting firmly? How does your backside feel against the chair? Your back?

Listen to the sounds around you. What can you hear in the background? Road noise? Birds? The sound of your breathing? Choose one sound and try to notice the details of the sound — the volume, the pitch, the gaps between the sounds. Notice if your mind starts to tell you stories about what you can hear, and, as best you can bring your mind back to focus on the details of the sounds themselves.

Now look around you and find a visual point on which to focus. It might be a plant leaf or a photograph on the wall. Closely notice the details of this point. Notice the shades of colour, the texture, the shape — how the sun falls on this spot. Maintain this focus as long as you can and try and notice the details that you might not have seen before.

Now, check your watch again. How long were you able to keep this up for? Three minutes? Five? It can be surprisingly hard to stop for ten minutes and become aware of our surroundings. How did you feel while you were doing this exercise? What was the state of your mind? Did you feel frustrated at being still or did you feel a sense of calm?

This focusing activity is just one example of the type of techniques that you might work on to master meditation. I have found that it does help in a wide range of situations where drawing your attention to the details of your surroundings can distract you from irritation, boredom or even pain. At the very least it can help you to become more aware of what is on your mind and how you are feeling physically — and take you away from your automatic train of thought — if only for a few moments. Meditation does take training and practice though. If you are interested in learning more, there are excellent books and courses around to get you started, and there are a few listed in the Appendix. I recommend having a go!

Exercise

For many men, exercise is their preferred way to reduce physical and mental stress. They feel comfortable with the approach and indeed exercise is generally associated with better psychological wellbeing.

However, there are many other good reasons to exercise if you have had a diagnosis of cancer or are close to someone who has. First, there is evidence that physical inactivity and being overweight are risk factors for not only getting some cancers but also doing less well after cancer. Second, many men who have prostate cancer are also at risk for heart or cardiovascular disease due to their age, as are their partners. So reducing your risk of other chronic diseases so you can enjoy your life together in good health makes sense.

Not doing any exercise and being physically inactive is unhealthy for anyone, but even more so for a man with prostate cancer. It is well established through large amounts of research that exercising most if not every day really improves physical and mental health for men with prostate cancer. So much so that men are being encouraged to exercise in the weeks leading up to any surgery to build their resilience. Exercising while on testosterone suppression or hormone-blocking treatment is also well established for reducing side effects such as fat gain and muscle and bone loss. Further on in the list of beneficial effects, exercise can improve urinary control and sexual function, reduce fatigue and tiredness, improve sleep, help with balance and reduce the risk of falls, and is associated with better thinking (cognitive ability) — all important things for enjoying a full and satisfying life after prostate cancer. There also is a relationship between physical activity and in particular vigorous exercise with improved prostate cancer survival.

While any exercise is beneficial, the latest Australian position statement on exercise medicine for cancer management recommends men with prostate cancer seek advice from an Accredited Exercise Physiologist to be assessed and prescribed a targeted exercise program for even greater effectiveness. Details about how to find this advice are included in the Appendix. You might hear your doctor or people in your health care team talk about this as exercise medicine, and so the point of seeing an accredited exercise physiologist is to get the exercise prescription right, from the get-go, and to adjust the prescription if needed, for example, if treatment or your personal concerns change.

Of course, we all know we should exercise more. The trouble is getting motivated to start, finding the time, choosing a way to exercise that you can practically stick to, and then keeping it up. A good way to start is to first think about how much you value your health and wellbeing and the things you are looking forward to in the future that you want to be physically well for. From this, you need to set goals for physical activity that match what matters most to you and then make a commitment to do this for *yourself*.

Key practical steps to exercise are to have a health check-up with your doctor before you take on a new exercise plan, and then get really good advice from an expert (such as an exercise physiologist) to make sure that the plan you have will get you where you want to go. Unguided exercise can be pretty hit or miss in terms of achieving results, and without good advice you are more likely to end with a strain or over-use injury that slows you down. In a way, what you want is the maximum benefit for the least effort — an efficient and targeted exercise plan that gets you where you want to go.

There are two different types of primary exercise you will want to aim for: strengthening (or resistance) exercise and aerobic exercise. Resistance exercise, using as examples weights or elastic bands, will build muscle and muscle strength where you need and want it most. Aerobic exercise will build your cardiovascular fitness and help with weight control. Getting a good balance of these two approaches will keep your body working at its best and also help keep you free from injuries. As a general rule, you need to exercise for twenty to sixty minutes at least three times a week to get a meaningful benefit. Higher intensity exercise is now seen as a very effective means of improving cardiovascular fitness. In practical terms, this involves exercising with a higher heart rate but perhaps for shorter periods (separated by 'recovery' bouts of lower intensity exercise).

The final point to make is that it can be easier to stick to an exercise plan if you have a friend or partner to exercise with. It just makes it more fun! As well, if you set exercise goals and share these with a friend or your partner, they can support and help motivate you to keep it up.

Activity

If you already meditate three days a week and are currently training to climb Kilimanjaro, then no activity work for you! On the other hand, if you are like most people and could do with a little less tension and a little more exercise, you need to set some goals.

Think about how you feel most of the time. Do you think you have room for improvement in the way you look after yourself? Use the checklist below as a start and prioritise which of these things you would most like to work on.

- Exercising more
- Feeling calmer
- Reducing my weight
- Feeling stronger physically
- Any other ways?

The next step is to draw up a plan of attack. Be clear about your goals first and the short and medium-term milestones you want to reach, and when you expect to get there. List the steps you will need to take to move towards these milestones, who and what you need to help you achieve these, and what barriers you might need to cross or deal with as you go. Consider that there are many different ways to help you achieve your goals. You might like to join a yoga or tai chi class, start walking with a friend, or just take some quiet space in each day to 'drop anchor' and calm your mind. Finally, pick a date to get started, tell your close friends or partners about your plan so they can keep a check on you, and go for it!

Remember, setbacks are normal, and watch yourself for unhelpful 'all or nothing' thinking. Most things that are worthwhile are effort, but if you never start, you most certainly will not get there.

Personal Stories

Following is a personal story from Charles about how he came to take up an exercise program to help with prostate cancer treatment side effects that has turned into a normal way of life for him and his partner. Jan and Gordon talk about how they use mindfulness and breathing techniques to manage stress. Roger talks about how he got into dragon boating and how this has enhanced his fitness and his social life. Patrick explains how he maintains his physical and psychological health through exercise, meditation and the pursuit of knowledge.

Charles

> I was diagnosed with an aggressive prostate cancer in 2011. I was 76 years of age at the time. Because of my age and also that I had had heart surgery in the past, my urologist and radiation oncologist suggested radiation therapy, both brachytherapy and external beam, and a six-month course of hormone-blocking injections. It was a big shock at the time, and I do think that is the biggest challenge, getting over that shock. In the end though, what can you do but take a positive outlook? I just thought: 'Alright then, I can't change it, so I will do my best to fix it and do what I can to get well'.
>
> The side effects of the hormone treatment were pretty tough. I put weight on around my girth, and that bothered me since I had always kept my weight steady. The hot flushes were the worse, five or six a night, and in the summer heat in the west that is hard going. It gave me new sympathy for what women go through in the menopause! The best tip I got was when my doctor referred me to an exercise program based at Edith Cowan University at their Health and Wellness Institute in Perth. I went along there and was assessed by the exercise physiology team. They looked at my bone density, my physical fitness, a really comprehensive check-up. From that, they worked out an exercise program suited to my individual needs. The

program they set me went for three months initially, it was in a small group of three people and included walking on a treadmill as well as a series of exercises involving weights. These included things such as lifting leg weights, step-ups, and shoulder and arm resistance exercises. We had to tinker with the program now and again though. I have arthritis, and after a while I just couldn't manage the dumbbells. The alternative we tried was a medicine ball which was terrific and enabled me to keep up my upper body exercises. Whenever there was a problem the exercise physiologist found a creative way to get around it. Once my plan was sorted out I was able to do the exercise program in my local gymnasium to cut down my travel, as I live in Freemantle. After six weeks, I went back to Edith Cowan to have the tests again and to check my progress and everything was improved! My bone density was better, my muscles had tightened up again, and I was much stronger. In fact, by the end of three months I had improved an old back injury to the point where I didn't need a walking stick anymore, so I was better than ever.

Apart from the physical benefits of the exercise program, I think it helps you mentally to be able to do something to help yourself. We did the program in a small group, so I made new friends, and the gymnasium is a pretty stimulating environment, lots of people to talk to and lots going on. It got me out of the house as well and really established clearly to me that I was not the only one going through this. That helped me a lot.

I have kept the exercise up even though I am now not on the hormone treatment. My wife has always been very supportive, we have been married now for 57 years, and she wanted to get involved as well. So we bought ourselves a treadmill and an exercise bike and some weights and we now do the routine at home, every day. It is pretty simple really. We also try and walk about two to three kilometres a day. You do have to be disciplined to keep it up, but it helps to do it together, and the benefits are well worth it. To keep well, this is one thing I can do.

Gordon

One of the hardest things I find is trying not to spend too much energy worrying about what might happen tomorrow.

My view is we need to live for today, but we also have to live with the understanding of the disease, which the doctors tell me is at the stage where I can't be cured. Knowing that makes a big difference to what you are doing. At the moment everything is fine, the path I am on right now is that I can basically do whatever I like and still enjoy it. There are times though when the thoughts come in, like when the Olympic games finished, is that the last Olympic games I will be able to watch? When those thoughts come in I get some sense of urgency, like I need to do this now because I might not be able to do it in the future. It's a case of also being aware of the situation I am in and asking myself if what I am doing has a point, or should I invest my energy elsewhere? Jan says I am a great procrastinator. She calls me 'Random Global' — I have a picture with 4000 things in it that I want to do, and prioritising these is hard! There are so many things out there to do, you move forward a little bit on this one and a little bit on that one, and some things get to completion, and others don't. That's probably the frustrating part for me is that I don't complete as many things as I should. But that doesn't stop me trying.

For de-stressing, the thing that is best for me at the moment is the breathing exercise. When I get into a situation that feels a bit tough, I do a two-minute breathing exercise, which is just a relaxation approach. I also try and focus on the now, the present, focus on what I am doing and move everything else away. When I get aches and pains or when a situation develops, and I am starting to feel stressed, I focus on what I am doing now, the very simple things, and what I am doing in this moment. It helps me to keep going and come out the other side in a positive state. I find the relaxation tapes help as well, being able to sit and listen and take your mind away. I really enjoy doing that although I haven't been doing this lately as much as I should.

Jan

I found out about mindfulness from a counsellor I was seeing at the Cancer Council Queensland. She mentioned that this course was coming up and asked would I be interested. It was an eight-week group course, I mentioned it to Gordon and asked if he wanted to come to, and he said why not, so that is how we got in.

For the first few weeks it was difficult. I guess I was concerned that Gordon was the only bloke in the room.In fact I was quite concerned and distressed for his sake. I could only imagine how I would have felt if I had been the only woman in a room full of men, so there was that to it. But he settled in about halfway through the course. By that stage it was almost genderless; there was only the odd occasion when we would roll our eyes at each other! The other thing we did was to make sure that after every mindfulness course we would go to dinner somewhere in town to some bohemian restaurant, so we always had something to look forward to afterwards. As it turned out, while we always enjoyed our dinners, we didn't really need to go to dinner afterwards because the sessions became more and more enjoyable. We began to really look forward to them. They were difficult in the first instance because the actual act of mindfulness is really hard at the start. All of us in the group were struggling. I guess what I am saying is that mindfulness is not an easy practice to learn after many, many years of letting your brain do whatever it wants to do, whenever it wants to do it. Probably up to week five it was a real struggle, after that, I stopped judging myself, and then it became a more enjoyable process.

The mindfulness exercise which I find the easiest is the one that involves part body scan, part listening and part feeling. For me to do fifty minutes of just scanning my body is torture and I find it really difficult. It is much easier for me to listen to what's going on outside and just enjoy the simple things like the sun on your body or the sounds around you.

Roger

I was diagnosed with prostate cancer just over nine years ago, which was pretty traumatic at the time. I had a great surgeon though, and he got me through it really. Then, about one year later my PSA started to rise, I went on hormone-blocking treatment, but again after about another year later the problem recurred. Luckily, there was a clinical trial, a vaccine trial actually, that my doctor found I was eligible for. Since then, between the trial and my hormonal therapy, I have kept really well.

One thing I do for myself is to keep very active. About four years ago I got into dragon boating. Dragon boating is great exercise, you actually use your stomach muscle or core strength more than your arms, and I can tell you that working out in a dragon boat four times a week gets you fit! I have always loved the water. When I was a baby my grandpa used to take me out netting for flounder, and I would play with the baby flounder in the bottom of the boat! I grew up in Hobart and was always on the water, fishing on the jetty, and rowing dinghies and sailing yachts on the Derwent River. So when a friend suggested dragon boating to me, it was a great fit. You also get to meet a lot of great people, from all walks of life, so from a social point of view it is brilliant as well as fun. There is also something really calming about being close to the water, a great mix.

About the time I took up dragon boating, I also decided to improve my diet, moving to more fresh fruit and vegetables. Over time I lost 20 kilograms in weight, so now I am a healthy weight for my height and age. The exercise also helps with the muscle wastage that you get from the hormone treatment, and the tiredness.

I do a lot of volunteering as well, and a lot of this is connected to exercise. I have been working with the Relay for Life program of the Cancer Council Queensland for many years, and in fact, in 2010 I was named the Relay for Life International Hero of Hope, one of only 13 at that time in the world. Relay for Life is a fundraising event that involves walking or running for 24 hours in teams. My aim now is to raise money with the hope I can save more than one life from cancer. This is all I do with my life now and I enjoy all the people I am involved with. I have the normal side effects from the hormone treatment, mostly tiredness and a bit of a dull head at times. I am used to these effects now and my way of coping is to keep busy, look after my overall wellness, and not pay these negative effects too much attention. I will be 70 this year and I am still standing up and enjoying life so I can't complain!

Patrick

I was 55 years old when I was diagnosed, and that's a good seventeen years ago now. My GP had been doing yearly blood tests on me as a regular check since I turn 50, and to be honest I never took much notice. Then one day out of the blue, his receptionist called and asked me to come in to see him, and then I got the news. That was the start of my journey. Fortunately, I was already a bit savvy about prostate cancer. I had a cousin who was 18 months post-surgery for prostate cancer and also a work colleague who had had treatment. This was just as well because the first urologist I saw was not at all helpful — poor manner and aggressive I thought. So I went on to get a second and third opinion, and by asking around and researching, I was able to make a good decision about my treatment approach and who I wanted in charge of my care. I had a radical prostatectomy, it all went well, and the post-operative care was great. I regained my continence very quickly, in the first week, and slowly over time my erectile function improved. Still not what it used to be but then as you age this happens naturally anyway.

It wasn't all a breeze though. I had trouble as a single man finding a support group where I could be open about my fears and concerns. I was really looking for guys who had been through the same experience. A big issue for me was trying to work out how to get back to being physically active the way I had been before. I couldn't find a road map for my overall physical recovery and I wanted to move forward. I had always been a serious rower and rowed in the Australian Masters Games. And I loved windsurfing. I wanted to know how I could get my strength back and what I could do. It was hard back then to find answers. Prostate cancer was less talked about and I felt quite alone.

In the end, through family and friends' support I went back to the gym and that was a great start. A friend introduced me to yoga, and this gave me the added benefit of finding a connection between my physical wellbeing and psychological health. I learnt to meditate, and over time to practice mindfulness. This helps me to feel calmer and to be more accepting of my life and the uncertainty about the future. My family shouted me some Pilates sessions to work on strengthening my abdominal core, and that was also very helpful for rebuilding my strength after having had major surgery. I swim now in stillwater beaches and find as I am doing my laps that I am able to connect with the environment, and so again, this has a relaxation effect that brings extra value to my quality of life.

I keep active now, not the same as before, but then I am getting older and this has meant I have had to adjust to my body changing. I used to feel quite envious sitting on the beach and watching the younger men kite surfing, and thinking, that would have been me, should have been me. I do still regret giving up windsurfing. But those feelings have lessened over time. I am an active learner about the natural world, astronomy, the 'big bang', I have a yearning for knowledge and I follow this. Understanding more about the universe and where I sit in it helps me feel more accepting of life transitions and change. I feel better about myself and am better able to cope with life challenges. I judge myself less.

For men being diagnosed now, my advice is be informed from both the medical and technical side of things as well as personal experience. Tap into the support and guidance that is around to help you make sense of things and make decisions you are comfortable with. Look after your physical and psychological health. The two go together like a horse and carriage. Commit to this. Try to accept the changes prostate cancer and ageing bring. You will not be weaker, just different.

As I look back 17 years to my prostate treatment, would I be as proactive in keeping up my mental and physical health as I have done? Would I have been more content to just let myself age and let life take its course? It is hypothetical, so there is no really true answer. But recovering from a life drama like prostate treatment, has I think spurred me on to more action than I might have taken. Can I look back and say 'out of a negative, a positive has happened!'? I think for me, and this is purely personal, I say yes. I am ready to get on with life.

Chapter 9

Solving Problems After Treatment

So, back to 'facing the tiger': If I can't fight or run, what can I do? Adopting a problem-solving approach is one good option.

Problem-solving is of course part of everyday life. We do it all the time, often with little focused thought. Some people are more efficient at solving problems than others, but most of us could probably do better at this with a more planned approach. After a prostate cancer diagnosis most men and their partners will at one time or another run into problems they haven't dealt with before. This is very unfamiliar territory for most people and it can feel a little overwhelming.

In this situation, using a more systematic approach to solving problems can help. In brief, this approach breaks the problem down into manageable chunks and helps you move forward towards an answer. A problem-solving approach can be applied to very practical problems, such as coping with treatment side effects, and also for emotional or relationship problems that are sometimes a bit harder to talk about or deal with straight up.

The first step is to be clear about what the problem is, so define the problem and find accurate information about the issue so that you understand why it has arisen and what it means. This might mean reading over cancer treatment booklets from a reputable source such as the Prostate Cancer Foundation of Australia or the Cancer Council, talking to your doctor or prostate care nurse, and meeting with and talking to other men who have also had prostate cancer or their partners who might have experienced this problem and be able to provide advice from a personal perspective.

From this, you will be able to generate different options or possibilities for dealing with the problem. The more alternative solutions you generate the better. The point is to come up with as many different ideas as possible.

Next, evaluate the pros and cons of each possible solution. This should include what help you might need and from whom, how confident you feel about each approach working for you, and from this, a preferred option should emerge.

Once you have a preferred option, then you can start on the plan. Your plan needs to be clear about the steps you will need to take and should have a timeline for each step. Finally, be clear about what success would mean for this problem and how you will evaluate for yourself how you have gone. As you go, though, be prepared to re-evaluate your plan and adjust or change it if it doesn't seem to be working for you. Having a flexible approach is crucial.

Here are some examples of how this approach could be applied to problems that are not unusual after prostate cancer treatment.

Example One: Fatigue and Getting Back to Work

Andrew is 58 years old. He works in the retail business and has been in this company for over five years. He has just received his last external beam radiation therapy session and is pretty happy to get to the end of that. After six weeks of radiation therapy he is feeling really tired. But even though he is tired most of the time and can get to sleep fairly easily, he finds he wakes up in the middle of the night, tosses and turns for an hour or two, before drifting back to sleep. And he wakes up tired. He is also on hormone-blocking treatments which his doctor says he will be for another ten months, and he feels he is losing condition and strength physically. He is starting back at work in two weeks and is wondering how he will cope.

Andrew actually has a number of concerns going on, and they are likely compounding each other:

- Tiredness.
- Insomnia or sleeplessness.
- Muscle loss as a side effect of hormone-blocking treatment.
- Worry about returning to work.

When Andrew reflects on all of these problems and which one is bothering him the most, it is the tiredness and poor sleep that gets the biggest tick. He feels that if he was less tired, he would feel more ready for the office and less anxious.

There are good reasons why Andrew feels tired. Tiredness or fatigue is a common side effect of radiation therapy and can be prolonged. Most patients will experience this, yet they often don't expect it and if they feel this way don't always tell their doctors about it. Hormone blocking agents can cause tiredness, so this is also in the mix. Finally, stress and worry can lead a person to feel tired. Having cancer is stressful.

A first step for Andrew was to talk to his family doctor about his tiredness as his main worry and get a clear explanation of the cause. He had been feeling that he was weak and should be more resilient, and so now he knows the facts he can stop blaming himself for not being up to the task. One of the best ways to work on tiredness and fatigue is exercise medicine. So Andrew's doctor refers him to an Accredited Exercise Physiologist (AEP) and gives him a Chronic Disease Management Plan so that he can obtain a Medicare rebate for up to five sessions. Andrew takes this up and sets a date for his first gym session.

Andrew gets tips for better sleep hygiene from his family doctor to try out as a first step for improving his disrupted sleep. Andrew is going to stop his afternoon naps, stay up a little later in the evening (until around 9 pm), cut down on alcohol during the week, and plans to stop drinking coffee in the afternoon. His new exercise program will make a difference as well, and he is going to try some relaxation breathing techniques before he goes to sleep and if he wakes in the night. His family doctor asks him to call back in four to five weeks and let him know how he is going.

Andrew meets his AEP at the gym the next week and starts an exercise program that will specifically target the effects of his hormone therapy as well as build his aerobic fitness. The plan is for weekly gym visits along with exercise at home.

Andrew also decides to contact two of his workmates to catch up. He had been avoiding people during treatment but now sees that it is time he reconnected. His mates were pleased to hear from him, and they make a time to meet up before he starts back at work. He also plans to call his manager and touch base, given he has been away for several weeks, and also to check on the possibility of a graded or gradual return to work if his fatigue continues to be a problem.

• • •

Reflecting on this story you can see the close interaction between what we do and how we feel. Tiredness and fatigue from treatment, compounded by sleep disturbance and a strategy of avoidance, were bundled up together and presented as a barrier for Andrew to get back to work and his usual way of life. There were real strategies though, actions that Andrew could take to address this. He just needed to be clear about the issues, get good advice, make a plan, and then commit to it. Keeping up good habits over time can be tough, so Andrew will need to plan ways to keep his motivation going, especially with his exercise program. Setting achievement goals and marking his progress and achievements as he goes will help, as well as getting support from his friends. A cheer squad helps! If he has setbacks, and most people will at some point, taking a problem-solving approach and resisting self-blame (it's pointless) will help Andrew get back on track. It is a life journey to develop good health habits, but an active approach pays real dividends for overall well-being.

Example Two: Solving Urinary Problems

Bill and Hillary are a couple from Sydney in their early sixties. They have been married for 15 years. Bill had a radical prostatectomy eight weeks ago and is still having problems with urinary control. He is wearing a pad all the time, and during the day has to change this at least three times. As a result, he is not going out of the house much, his partner Hillary is irritable about them staying home all of the time, and Bill is feeling frustrated with the pace of his recovery. Because of the urinary leakage they haven't tried to have sex and both Bill and Hillary find it hard to talk about this.

If you reflect on what is happening for Bill and Hillary there are actually *at least* six pieces or 'chunks' to this problem:

- Urinary leakage
- Being housebound
- Feeling stressed about recovering from treatment
- Not feeling close as a couple
- Not having sex
- Having difficulty communicating

It is important to be clear about all the chunks in this problem because although they all seem related, each of these issues needs different strategies and all involve both Bill and Hillary. Fortunately, Bill and Hillary eventually decide they need to use a problem-solving approach to move forward.

Considering each of these issues, they decide to start with urinary leakage. By reading up on the subject and talking to Bill's surgeon they know that the reason this can happen is damage at the time of surgery to the tissues and nerves that control passing urine. Understanding that this is a problem that usually resolves over time helps, and knowing that if Bill does regular pelvic floor exercises for his muscles he can speed up the repair process provides a basis for a plan. Bill decides to go to a physiotherapist to get help with learning how to do pelvic floor exercises. Hillary decides she needs to learn them as well. Since the babies and the menopause, her urine control has not been great either!

Bill goes to a local prostate cancer support group meeting and he is able to borrow a copy of a self-help book on pelvic floor exercises from a chap he meets there. At the support group Bill meets other men who have also experienced this problem and he learns that it is pretty common to be still using a few pads a day at this stage. He is reassured to find out that he will probably be down to one pad a day in a month or so and that most men are dry by six months. The men he talks to also have great practical tips for managing this problem when out and about. He now feels less like he is the only one with this problem and more hopeful about the future. It is a relief! He has found a map of where the public toilets are in the city centre and he feels confident enough to make a plan with Hillary to go to the movies together next weekend.

Hillary and Bill decide to make a time to talk about how they are coping as a couple. They set aside a morning and share with each other how they have been feeling of late. Both Hillary and Bill agree they want to get back to being closer and more like they were before the cancer. As a first step, they agree that more hugs and touching and physical closeness, but with no expectation of sex, is needed. Bill wants to get his urine control a bit better before they try at sex, even though they both know that urine leakage during sex is not at all harmful. They do want to get sex back on track in the future though so Bill makes an appointment with his doctor for both him and Hillary to find out about what options are available for helping Bill get an erection. Both Bill and Hillary are aware that working on Bill having regular erections earlier rather than later is part of good 'penis health' after prostate cancer treatment.

In the meantime, Hillary books a weekend away at the beach for her and Bill and buys an erotic book and some massage oil, just in case they get in the mood for some extra closeness. The main plan though includes long walks on the beach and relaxation. Hillary has been doing some meditation classes to help her relax and de-stress, and Bill has agreed to give it a go (or at least try the breath control exercises) while they are on their weekend away.

• • •

If you look over this hypothetical story (although I have known many men and their partners who have experienced these actual problems) you can see that each chunk of the problem needed different strategies, even though the issues were all related and seemed to stem from the urinary problems. Bill and Hillary took the time first to be clear about the problem and talk about it together. Their next step was to get more information about what they could do about it and then talk this through to develop an agreed preferred approach. They now will need to put this into action, and if needed, revise the plan as they go along.

Taking your time with a well-considered plan will help you to not miss important opportunities to make things work better for you. Involving your partner or a support person, like a son or daughter or close friend, in the making of the plan will help make sure you are both pulling together and working as a team.

Activity

In your note pad or journal make a list of the main problems that are worrying you right now. Do this separately on your own and then share these with your partner. Do you have some problems that you both are concerned about and could work on together? Are there things worrying your partner that you were unaware of?

Next, prioritise this list using number 1 for the problem that is most important to you right now, 2 for the next most important, and so on.

Pick off your top three priorities and ask yourself if you understand clearly how this problem has arisen. If you need more information about the problem, make a decision to find out more.

Once you feel you are well informed, generate a list of possible actions you could take to help with each priority and consider which actions you feel comfortable doing and most confident about. Think about who can help you with this and what extra support you might need, and what milestones you want to reach and when.

Now you have a plan you can move into action, but remember that if all does not go the way you planned or hoped it is okay to reconsider and revise the plan.

Personal Stories

Below is a personal story from Norman about how he approached problems he faced after prostate cancer treatment, and this included getting outside support with the help of his son Tristan when things got very tough. Gerry talks about how he was a bit too chilled out after treatment, and Graham shares how a very tough time turned around once he got the right advice.

Norman

> Being diagnosed in late 2007 was a real shock. The prognosis was challenging and required a different approach to treatment. The best option was considered to be brachytherapy, followed by external beam radiotherapy, and hormone treatment for a few months before the brachytherapy. The hormone therapy was awful; it brings about a huge loss of energy and makes working accurately challenging. Simply going for a walk was difficult. The hot flushes happened at any time and could be embarrassing. I knew I had to try to understand this cancer and the treatment to make some sense of it all, and thereby accept and know what lay ahead. This I did using many sources such as the Internet, discussion with health professionals, and contact with the Brisbane Prostate Cancer Support Group. Gradually I felt I had built a picture that reassured me.
>
> The big day arrived, and I was very confident that the next two parts of the treatment would be a breeze. I knew all about this stuff! In fact, the brachytherapy went very well, really just as expected. There are a few things that are confronting, as with any surgery. A few days after the brachytherapy I started daily external beam radiation. At first this seemed to go well until my mind started to 'spin-out' with thoughts of radiation burn, the accuracy of the

beam, the challenge to my masculinity, and the thought that I may die before my wife.

I was still at work, so medical appointments were either early morning or late afternoon. You need to have a full bladder for each treatment. This added to my desperation until my wife suggested timing the start of hydration to arrive on the treatment table full and bursting, but avoiding accidents. I always needed a pit stop afterwards and still had the occasional accident on the table. Even though the treatment staff told me 'Mate that's all part of it, happens all the time, don't worry about it', I did worry about it! I was not coping with things, and I needed help. I took time off work, as that had become difficult. My iPod was loaded with calming music to help me relax before and during treatment. I changed appointments to mid-morning or mid-afternoon. These changes gave slight relief, but the issues were getting harder to avoid.

My son Tristan had been making sure that everything was going well but from the background. He could see that things were difficult for me, which impacted on my wife's concerns, as she was driving me to many appointments, and making sure I was progressing. He picked up on the fact that I needed some outside help to try to calm down and make sense of things. My son has always been very supportive of both of us. He never tries to run the show. Rather, he will look at situations and gently suggest some ideas. He believes in getting the right help and finding out how to source it. One of his friends knew a psychologist with a practice close to us. Between the two of them getting things happening, I had a very rewarding time making some sense out of my anxiety and somewhat irrational thoughts. This continued for a period with another counsellor. While it is hard to sit down with a complete stranger and lay out your innermost issues, it becomes less so as you work through what you choose to change, and is in fact very rewarding.

My son and I have become much closer in recent times, in terms of expressing appreciation and love for one another. Once he had reached sixteen such things seemed past history. But now a good man-hug and a brush cheek kiss are so welcome for both of us.

I have learnt a lot from my cancer journey. I have changed the way I live, interact with others, and now enjoy every moment of my life. Learning to meditate to calm the body, mind, and soul is satisfying. Living in the moment and savouring what is happening right now is my aim. While not always easy, sitting having coffee in a sunny spot, hearing the birds, feeling a slight breeze, or the smell of a freshly baked cookie grabs me now. Just as does the crackle of an open fire on a winter night, the smell of a barbecue, happy conversation and the clinking of glasses, and time with friends.

It is important to respect yourself and have the courage to be yourself. Life throws some unpleasant things at us. At dark times, take a tool which you have in your tool belt, apply it and surprise yourself.

Tristan

I couldn't believe it when Dad was diagnosed with prostate cancer. It didn't seem fair. Mum and Dad approached Dad's diagnosis as a team, and Dad initially approached the whole situation with calm confidence. He seemed confident in the treatment and in his medical team, and he even laughed off some of the more unpleasant aspects of the Brachytherapy treatment — including what we referred to as the porcupine stage!

It all changed when Dad started hormone therapy and radiotherapy. The confidence vanished and was replaced with fatigue, doubt and increasing despair. At first, I thought it was a side effect of the hormone treatment. He was depressed and was obsessing about his treatment. Then Dad refused to attend radiotherapy treatment one day. He could not face it anymore. It was a difficult time for all of the family.

While I was shocked and upset by the situation and the stark realisation of mortality — I also experienced it as a time of transition. To this point, my parents had been the strong ones — the carers. It felt very much like it was now my turn to assume the role of the strong one, the carer, while Dad was ill. I don't recall experiencing doubt or resentment — it just seemed like the right thing to do at a difficult time. In the words of the singer-songwriter John Mellencamp — 'There is nothing more sad or beautiful than generations changing hands.'

I was fortunate at that time to have a housemate who was studying psychology and developing a specialisation in crisis counselling. He was an excellent sounding board and a great friend. I discussed Dad's situation with him, and we identified a psychologist who could help him. I approached the topic gently with Dad — he was very wary of any medical treatment and did not, I think, have the awareness at that time that he was experiencing psychological trauma. I floated the idea and left it for Dad to consider. He agreed to meet the psychologist and to have an initial discussion. He did this on his own as I recall, but with Mum's support.

I am proud of the way in which Dad embraced counseling, which was explained to him as a simple kit of tools for Dad to use when faced with stressful situations. He has grown enormously as a person as a result, and we have grown far closer as father and son. Dad has continued to develop himself, to read, to meditate, and to share his experiences and learn from others.

Mum passed away in 2011. It was extraordinarily sad, but the way in which Dad approached this stressful time, this fundamental change in his life, was nothing short of inspiring. About a month after Mum passed away, I asked Dad how he was going. He said to me, 'I'm living in the moment. So many friends are asking me to meet them, to have dinner, to catch up — I've just decided I am going to say yes to them all.'

Gerry

I was diagnosed in 1998 and had a radical prostatectomy. My first concern was, am I going to survive any treatment? I had a suspicion about my heart, so I went through the process of being diagnosed with a heart condition then an angiogram then angioplasty. So I had to recover from that first. I didn't know until a few weeks before the surgery what I was going to do. It was an uncertain time; there was lots of talk of new therapies coming out from some of the centres in the United States, so it was confusing and a time of great turmoil. Slowly but surely I came to realise that I needed to understand an awful lot more, really understand how good these statistics actually were compared to what they were saying. There was always more to it than the statistics led you to believe.

Then, when I was in Sydney visiting my granddaughters, I was on the train, and there was a sign about a prostate cancer support group there. Believe it or not, at that time I had not even checked to see if there was one in Queensland where I live. So I gave them a phone call and they were a really good mob! Three guys — one had had radiation, one surgery and one guy was on watchful waiting. They spent an afternoon with me. It was wonderful. I figured out from that conversation what I needed to know about most and how I could find out more.

During the five months which had passed since diagnosis, my PSA had gone up from 6.5 to 11 — clearly, something had to be done. By the time I had made up my mind about treatment, I thought: 'Well I am stuck with whatever the outcome so I had better get on with it!' I had made up my mind that whatever the outcome of treatment was, I was going to live with it and accept it and go on from there.

My approach after treatment was to work out what strategies I could apply to make things easier to get over. What I didn't do, and what I should have done, was set myself a goal. Coming up to the end of my accrued sick leave after two months, I decided I had better go back to work. At that time I was still on a couple of pads a day. Once I paid attention to this with my exercises very soon I was dry. If I had set myself a goal earlier, I would have reached that point sooner. I had decided I wasn't going to get uptight about it no matter what and so I had let this slide. I was just a lazy boy!

Fourteen years on now, I guess the main thing that I worry about is my PSA tests. There is always that chance that my PSA will effect a sudden change, but at my age we are looking at death from other causes, so you need to keep it in perspective. My main message to men now is when you have a problem to solve you are really looking at making a decision. You have to decide if you are going to act, and then if yes, choose your approach. Make sure that you understand the problem and break it down into steps. You've got to consider what's important and what needs to be dealt with first, and consider carefully why that's important as against the other things in life that are important to you.

Graham

I was initially diagnosed by my family doctor in 2009 and had a radical prostatectomy. All I wanted was to have the cancer removed, just get rid of it. It was all very matter of fact at the time. One minute I had a prostate and the next I didn't. My surgeon did actually say to me one day when we were talking: 'We are removing that many prostates at the moment that it is just like picking pineapples.'

I knew of absolutely nobody else who had had their prostate out, so I was totally alone. I didn't know where I could go to for support.

My major problem after surgery was urinary incontinence. I was told that some men suffer from some form of incontinence after a radical prostatectomy, but mine was just terrible. A few days after the operation and prior to leaving the hospital a physiotherapist told me about pelvic floor exercises, which I didn't even know existed until then. Then as I left hospital, I was handed some pads and that was it. I had very little knowledge about incontinence, and now I look back I don't know that I researched it enough. I guess I expected the doctor to sort it all out for me.

For two years I struggled with the incontinence, saw three physiotherapists, but the best I got down to was five pads a day. Everywhere I went I had to take pads, even on a trip to Turkey! My wife was fabulous about it. She would say: 'It's only wee.' But it's not the fact that it's only wee, it's the fact that you are wet all the time and your skin is wrinkly and you can't get dry. It's just so demoralising. In retrospect, I think that it made me a bit aggressive. I would get really angry at other people for complaining about things they should be grateful for. I was thinking: 'Why was it me that had this?' I have never been a person that was a 'why me' type, but it certainly made me one at the time.

Then through a support group I learnt about a surgical treatment for this problem — a sling, and it worked! It is absolutely amazing — in hospital overnight and now completely dry!

I decided to also get a penile implant to get over the erectile problems I was experiencing. I had tried everything for this. I tried the tablets and they gave me headaches. I found the injections didn't suit me either. I am a bit funny with needles, so to decide I was going to have sex then take time out and inject myself and come back — that just wasn't for me.

Honestly, once I got the implant and the sling my whole mindset completely changed. I told the doctor that did the implant that I remember as a young fellow my dad would say that you really feel good if you have a few beers in the fridge but you don't have to go and drink it. Another friend says they are always comfortable if they have chocolate in the fridge. These are the two things that stay in my mind with the implant. You mightn't use it for a week or two, but you feel bloody good that you can access it.

It's a mindset thing, and you don't understand a lot of this until after the event. You cope, and then you think how did I get through that? But you just do. My mind ticks over all the time about it, but once you are fixed, you get much more relaxed about it all. I am almost proud now that I have an implant and a sling.

I know many men may not experience the problems that I experienced, but whatever problems they do experience my message is: 'Don't give up, there is an answer.' I am happy to say I had wonderful support from my wife and friends. Men tend not to talk about their health issues. I have learnt to be more open. If someone is available to listen or help — take the opportunity!

Chapter 10

Getting Unstuck

Definition: freed or loosened from being fastened

In life, we all have our stories. About how we grew up, the good and bad things that have happened to us, the people who helped and the people who hindered, the things we are proud of, and what we might regret. Woven together this becomes our story or *narrative* about who we are, how our life generally plays out, what we hope for, what we strive for, what we expect, and what we need to live.

Sometimes though, life throws us a curveball and we find the narrative we have been working with doesn't seem to help us, and we can't seem to move forward or get over the speed bump. In other words, we get stuck. If you are feeling 'stuck' this might mean that you need a different approach to how you are looking at your cancer diagnosis and your future and how you sit in the world. This counts for men with prostate cancer and their partners equally.

Perhaps you are feeling anxious a lot of the time and are finding it hard to relax and feel easy in your skin. You might be living with a sense of grief and loss that is weighing you down — or worrying a lot of the time about the future and what it could hold. Maybe you are angry or annoyed more than you would like or feel that your relationships are not working as well as they might. These two things might be linked or closely connected. Or you are feeling a need for more direction in your life or a shift to a different purpose.

But first, you need to decide if you are really up for change and what that might mean, and what yearnings or past grievances you might need to let go of. This starts with awareness and reflection about your story or narrative — how you got to this point in life and what that narrative means to you. Doing the same thing repeatedly will generally lead to the same outcome. Is your current approach serving you well? Are you up for considering change? If yes, the first step is awareness.

Activity — Awareness

Set aside some time when you won't be interrupted. Find a comfortable place to sit where your body is well supported and relaxed. Start by building awareness of your breath. Gently place your hands on your belly. If you feel relaxed to do so, close your eyes. Breathe slowly to a count of four for each in-breath and each out-breath. Notice the breath coming into your body through your nose, the temperature of the air as you draw this into your body. Notice how your belly expands as you breathe in and relaxes back as you breathe out. Maintain this focus on your breath and direct your attention to this sensation.

Now start to notice other parts of your body and how

they feel. The soles of your feet and what they are placed upon, the pressure you feel there. Notice your posture and whether it is tight or loose. Gently move your shoulders and check for tension in your neck. Notice how your facial muscles are feeling, is your brow relaxed? Is your jaw tight or loose?

As you are doing this, your mind might wander to the worries of the day or the jobs and tasks you have to do and that are on your mind. Notice these thoughts and the feelings that come with them and how these thoughts affect your body tension. These thoughts and feelings are not in and of themselves good or bad; they just are what they are. Notice them, be aware of them, and now gently direct your attention back to your breath.

Now listen to the sounds you can hear around you. This might be traffic noises, or birds, wind in the trees, household noises. This is where you are right now, in the present.

So now in the present moment, turn to your heart and your head. What changes are you looking for in how you sit in the present. What would this mean for you? What words describe how this would look and feel?

When you are ready, focus again on counting in for four and out for four on each breath, and then open your eyes and jot down the feelings and thoughts you became aware of, and the changes that you are looking for in your present moment or situation.

The next step is to consider more deeply what is going on for you right now.

Activity — Where I am right now

Feelings

Write down the feelings you often experience that are difficult or uncomfortable to sit with.

How do you express those feelings to yourself and to those close to you?

Thoughts

Write down some thoughts that tend to come with these difficult or uncomfortable feelings.

What do you think might be the source of these thoughts? Do you treat these thoughts as if they are absolute truths — as facts that are certain and can't be changed?'

Is there a way you can talk or speak about these thoughts and see them as just thoughts? Look at them from a distance as if they were a story you had been told a long time ago.

As a next step, reflect with self-compassion how you would describe your life as it is right now.

Activity: Who am I?

If you were able to look at yourself as if you were a bystander to your life as it is right now, what would you see?

What advice would you give to yourself if you were your own best and trusted friend? Speaking to yourself as a compassionate adviser, what would you say?

Making Choices

How we live is up to all of us. Life will have delivered highs and lows, successes and losses. Rarely is this all good or all bad. It is our rich tapestry, it is our story or narrative, and we can become fused or glued to the past and our expectations of the future as if it is the only possible reality. We can get stuck in our past thoughts, feelings and behaviours and our expectations that this is all there is or can be. But how you experience the world and those around you *can* change into the future. Dwelling on the past is not likely to lead to change. Living in the present can lessen the burden of the past, and deciding to make changes for the future brings with it possibilities. No one is perfect, none of us. So accepting that and letting go of 'what ifs' and 'I should have' or 'might have' can be very freeing. This is about opening up to possibility, dropping self-blame, suspending judgement of ourselves and those around us, and responding to what we see and experience in new ways. Small changes can make important differences in how closely we connect with people who are important to us, and in how we walk into the future with ourselves in a spirit of self-compassion — being the self that we want to be, connecting with others the way we want to.

Activity — Where I want to be

What are the key areas of my life and how I am in the present that I would like to change? What do I hope for?

What thoughts or feelings are holding me back that would I need to step aside from to give myself a chance for change?

Trying out Change

Change is hard. Most of us tend to avoid it. A good place to start is to think of some small steps or actions towards how you want your life to be and set yourself up with these as experiments you can try. For example, if you have relationships that you would like to deepen and appreciate more, what might be an action you could take towards this? Perhaps there are activities you have always felt would be fun and rewarding but that you have avoided because of embarrassment or fear or never managing to find the time. Maybe you haven't felt you had earned the chance for change or something new or better. Make a list of things you have always wanted to try and select five to start with. Think of this as an experiment for acting and feeling differently. Lean in. Try saying yes.

Activity — Starting change

List five new activities or behaviours you would like to try; for example, meeting up with a good friend you haven't seen for some time; listening again to the music you most loved in your younger years or enjoying a good movie. Look for a short course on a topic you have always wanted to know more about. It's your list — what would expand your life?

Now schedule each of these activities to try out over the next six weeks. Commit yourself 100%. No self-evaluation or criticism is allowed. This is an experiment for you in widening out your range and view of what is possible in your life.

Personal Stories

Below is a personal story from Graeme about the setbacks and challenges he experienced from his prostate cancer diagnosis and after his partner died, and how he made a choice to open up to new experiences and reconnect with his community and his family in new ways.

Graeme

I was 47 years old when I was diagnosed with what turned out to be quite an advanced prostate cancer. My partner and I had recently moved so we had a new family doctor, and when I mentioned in passing that I had some problems with needing to pass urine frequently at night, he did an exam and felt some bumps and lumps that didn't seem right. I do have a family history of prostate cancer, my father and grandfather, so I guess this was already on the cards for me. I was sent to a urologist for a biopsy, and when the doctor phoned me at work to tell me I had cancer, I just went into shock. My colleagues said I went white. It's news you never really expect or want to hear. I was recommended for external beam radiation therapy and was happy to move rapidly on to getting treatment. I wanted to take action and felt while I was getting treatment I was fighting it, doing something.

I think I managed treatment well. I worked for most of it, would finish work at 3 pm, go to treatment, then home to rest and back to work the next day. My work manager was really supportive so that towards the end of treatment when I found the tiredness and fatigue were getting me down it was no problem to go on sick leave until it was over. Twelve months later though my PSA started to rise, and that was a setback. The doctor suggested we could watch and wait, but I wanted treatment. I didn't want this spectre on my shoulder. So I went on a course of hormone-blocking treatments — still in the game, fighting it. Of course, the hormone blockers have side effects; hot flushes were common. I managed to cope by changing how I felt about them — in my head they were 'power surges', treating the cancer and ultimately helping me.

The other effect though was psychological. I found I was feeling disengaged, almost like a spectator to life. This went on for some time until I recognised that I had mild depression. Once I understood that I felt relieved, I was normal. From this point onward I felt ready to again get on again with life.

However, life had more to throw at me. My partner of 18 years, Jess, died. I was devastated. I was lost in a deep sense of grief and loss. I realised then that I had become disconnected from my community and I needed to reach out. I had never had a strong belief in myself, but I had to summon up my courage and make myself do things. I needed to 'get a life'. A key step for me was to join a choir. As a child, I had played the piano, so I know music, and I have a strong voice with a wide range from second bass to tenor. I tried out and was able to join the Sydney Gay and Lesbian Choir, and later the University of Sydney Graduate and Chamber Choir. For me, this was transformative. There is a deep beauty in music that most of us can relate to, and the experience of being in a choir where you create music and are able to move people through music is marvellous. Being part of that creative process and the difference you can make to people's lives is deeply rewarding. The richness of tone that is created in harmony is an incredible thing. I am not sure if it is an addiction or a passion, or maybe it is both!

I also changed career and retrained as a licenced conveyancer. I decided to do this after a flash of insight when I was on holiday in Montreal for a choir performance. I was sitting on the banks of the St Lawrence River when I thought to myself, you have more to do. It is never too late to strike out in new ways that work for you.

I reconnected with my community through community celebration events like the Gay Games. This also helped me to heal. And my family were important, my brother and cousins and my aunt who were there for me. You need to open yourself up.

I think for men diagnosed now, remember it is your journey. You need to stand up for yourself and take back control, take back your life. Be informed so you know what is going on. A lot of the time you only hear one-third of what you are told so take a support person to important medical consultations. Reach out to support groups. Hearing the stories of others is immensely helpful and then you can see that you are not alone. Someone will be there to listen to your story. Give them a chance.

Chapter 11

Grace Under Fire

In his classic book, *The Old Man and the Sea*, Ernest Hemingway famously said that 'the definition of courage is grace under fire'. Whenever I read this quote I always think of all the men and women I have seen face cancer, taking what is thrown at them, and enduring. This takes courage, every day. Not only do people endure and move step by step and purposefully through this illness experience, they also often find new meaning in their social connections, their relationships and the world around them, take on new challenges in life, and sometimes develop a new way of being in the world.

Many people do say after cancer that although they would not wish this experience on anyone, least of all themselves, they have found benefits in their lives as a result. They also talk about the 'goal posts shifting', where what matters to them now is somewhat different and that their priorities have changed. The experience of cancer can be life-altering in ways other than the physical, and for some, can produce positive outcomes in unexpected ways.

Searching for Meaning

Asking 'why me' and wondering how it is that you or your partner came to be facing prostate cancer is a pretty common response. Cancer is not fair. It strikes people from all walks of life and backgrounds, and living a healthy, pure and honest life does not make you bullet-proof. A threat to life can lead you to wonder about the meaning of life and if 'this is it'. People sometimes ask themselves: 'What sort of person do I want to be? What sort of relationships do I want with others, and what do I want my life to be about?'

There are many philosophical traditions, Western and Eastern, that deal with this question: 'What is the meaning of life and what is the meaning of *my* life?' Some people find their religious or spiritual faith helpful and others find reflection, self-questioning and the seeking of knowledge an approach that leads to acceptance and strength. This is a personal and very individual path to walk, and there is no one right way to consider what having had cancer or loving someone who has had cancer, means to you. It is your journey.

It is important to note that some people do not see their diagnosis as a life-changing experience. For them, cancer is just another hurdle in life to manage and overcome as soon as they can with the resources they have available. For many others, the cancer experience leads them to re-evaluate how they view themselves and the world around them. These are the people who often report positive life changes after struggling with their cancer and treatment.

Finding the Good

If the goalposts shifted for you after a diagnosis of prostate cancer, you might have found that some aspects of your life have changed in a positive way. This is often called 'benefit-finding', which is pretty self-explanatory, or 'post-traumatic growth', which is a little more obscure. Both of these terms refer to when a traumatic event, such as a cancer diagnosis, shakes a person's world up to the point that they find themselves re-evaluating their life direction, personal priorities, relationships and future goals. This is an introspective and reflective process that can lead to a sense of personal growth, and for some people, decisions to change aspects of their lives. Post-traumatic growth is not confined to the experience of cancer; it can include the experience of war, loss of a loved one, road trauma or accidents. Any trauma where a person has experienced high levels of emotional distress and a threat to either their own wellbeing or the wellbeing of people close to them can lead to personal growth. Post-traumatic growth is its own universe in the sense that this positive aspect of change appears to be a separate outcome from the negative. The positive and negative don't cancel each other out, they co-exist.

A common way post-traumatic growth is expressed by people affected by cancer is that they now pay more care and attention to their loved ones and important personal relationships. Alternatively, sometimes a person might find their cancer is the tipping point that leads them to break off a relationship that perhaps has not been right for them for some time. Other people find they develop a new and deeper level of compassion for others and might take up volunteer work for a good cause or try and help others whenever they can. This compassion includes where a person finds within them forgiveness and kindness towards themselves, as well as towards others.

The courage or daring to try new challenges is another way people experience post-traumatic growth. Think of the people you know who have had cancer who take up marathon runs, walks or cycle trips to raise funds for cancer research as well as to challenge themselves physically. Dragon boating, mountain climbing, motorcycle riding, the list goes on. Many of the men and women who contributed their personal experiences about prostate cancer to this book have found their lives changed in these ways after cancer, and even just being prepared to share your story in this way is an act of courage.

Another way that people diagnosed with cancer or their loved ones express post-traumatic growth is by reporting a newfound sense of personal strength. This fits with that old saying 'what doesn't kill you, only makes you stronger'. Often people will comment that it wasn't until they were pushed did they realise how much they could deal with. Realising that you can cope with cancer may help you realise that you can cope with any of the challenges that life throws at you.

People who have been diagnosed with cancer often report that their priorities have now shifted. We can all become bogged down in the routine of life — work, paying the bills, commuting. Sometimes it takes something big to awaken us to all the possibilities that life has to offer. After struggling with cancer, some people may decide to spend more time with family and friends and less time at work, and some may decide to pursue life-long dreams that had previously been put on hold. This does not mean that everyone has or even needs to have this type of reaction to their cancer. Just getting through treatment and back to your usual life can be challenging enough.

Rebuilding Your Identity

After prostate cancer, who exactly are you? A person who has had prostate cancer or who loves someone who does? A cancer victim? A cancer survivor? A cancer patient?

Part of recovery is being comfortable with yourself, just as you are, at each stage of your recovery or role as a carer; and for men being okay with the parts of you that may have changed physically. For men who have had prostate cancer, the effects of treatment challenge sexual confidence in a way that hits to the core. It can be shattering to your masculinity and view of yourself as a man. Many men have told me rebuilding the masculine and sexual part of themselves is an ongoing 'work in progress'. As well, finding out you have cancer makes it hard to keep acting as if you are invincible, which is a typical 'blokey' attitude to the world and their health in particular. Feeling vulnerable about your health as well as your masculinity in this way is a tough road. Knowing that you are not alone helps. Talking about how this feels either to your partner or to other men who have also experienced prostate cancer can help you work this through to find a sense of coherence and rebuild your confidence.

After being diagnosed with cancer, some people are thrust into positions of role models in their circle of friends and their community. Others willingly take up raising awareness and funds for cancer research and offering support to others. Being diagnosed with cancer can open up a new network of friends, activities and events, and a new identity based on being a cancer survivor. Joining community groups and even taking part in research are just some of the ways that people feel like they can contribute and give back, as well as gain a sense of belonging with others who understand.

I know many people who proudly and often will say 'I am a cancer survivor', and for them, this means being strong, resilient and fearless. Others feel that they do not want to define themselves by their cancer, and see it more as an experience they have moved past. Again, neither way is right or wrong. What is important is to feel strong and confident about yourself and who you are now.

If you have faced the tiger, you know what it means to journey through struggle and difficulty, and this journey belongs to you.

Personal Stories

Below is a personal story from Peter about the challenges he took on after his prostate cancer and how this has influenced his life.

Peter

> As I talked about earlier (Chapter 2) the diagnosis, treatment and side effects of a radical prostatectomy in 1996 at age 52, left me reeling and searching for answers. My life suddenly deteriorated from being a healthy, fit, in-control, positive individual to one that was desperate, experiencing certain body-symptoms out of control, seriously depressed, bordering on suicidal and harbouring an exceedingly dark, repressed view of the world and the future.
>
> Once I'd made up my mind that I was not going to give up on myself, I reasoned I would need to understand the

process I was going through. This was achieved in several ways.

Firstly, gaining the assistance and support of other men who were travelling the same road was imperative.

At this level, we shared personal information and knowledge, developing strength as we empathised with each other. This was reinforced by attending lectures from health professionals of all disciplines involved with cancer and its side effects. Plus reading, studying, talking and asking — it was a time for coming out of 'our cave', regrouping and approaching the fight with this enemy as you would any battle.

As males, our lives have generally been programmed on autopilot, fulfilling stereotypes and traditional agenda roles placed on us by society. For the most part, we didn't mind or have any need to question this — the system worked well, allowing us to gain what we thought was high satisfaction out of life.

Until suddenly, something breaks down, and our expectations of life can't be fulfilled. It is particularly traumatic for men if the breakdown compromises our ability to work, to provide for ourselves and our family, and to have sex. (Prostate cancer can jeopardise all of these). At a time like this, it is important to contemplate some universal truths. What is a male? What is sex, and how important is it really? And the deeper ones: What is life? Is there a purpose to it? Relationships? God? Happiness? The list of unanswered questions goes on.

This process of readjustment takes time. It is really a search for a new reality — to work out how to redefine yourself, to rebuild a new self-image.

As tough as it seems, illness can provide us with the capacity to gain some new insights and wisdom, to cut through the nonsense and sham. There is no one answer to allow us to achieve this. Everybody will have different strategies to cope with their losses. Basically, cancer enables us to think about what's important and to prioritise things in our life. Seven years after my diagnosis and treatment, I felt the need for a sense of closure, to celebrate my new life. I was now nimble again and had developed purpose. I would climb Mt. Kilimanjaro — at almost 6,000m, the African continent's highest peak.

Why climb a mountain to prove anything? Most people would consider the exercise to be irrational. Perhaps, on one level, I see some symbolism of the uphill climb cancer survivors must face and overcome. On another level, it was a chance to measure myself, to balance the depressing threat to my life from cancer with elation for living. After a 60km climb through tropical jungle, hot, stifling but beautiful rainforest, to moorlands, alpine desert and finally, glaciers, ice and snow in sub-zero temperatures, I reached the summit on St. Valentine's Day, 2003.

This was a triumph and satisfied me for some years. However, I had now learned to appreciate life from a larger perspective. Life on earth started 3.8 billion years ago — I had been given one sliver of it to savour. I would live it passionately — I would climb another mountain, higher than Kilimanjaro. In December 2009, at age 66, I began climbing Mt. Aconcagua. At 6959m, the highest peak outside the Himalayas, Aconcagua soars out of the Andes in Argentina.

After eight days, we became trapped by a blizzard fifteen hundred metres below the summit. We were three weeks into the climbing season which had been marked by terrible storms. In that time, of 70 climbers who had attempted the summit, only 5 had succeeded, one of them perishing on the day before our group started for the top.

This news was highly distressing, adding to my fears. At this stage, I was seriously exhausted. I hadn't expected the continuing freezing conditions — minus 30 degrees — and was having trouble sleeping. My hands had been slashed by lifting sharp-edged rocks to keep our tents stable in the high winds, creating difficulty holding utensils to feed and look after myself.

While here, I was subject to an interesting phenomenon. We were advised not to go outside at night to urinate; it was too cold. The correct technique is to kneel inside the tent and deftly pee into a container. I didn't feel confident of achieving this, so I braved the elements outside. Expecting the scene to be black, I was shocked to see the landscape flooded with a burning silver light. The stars and moon were so close and unhindered by the atmosphere; they totally blazed. The Southern Cross was on fire right above me. In an intense physical and emotional experience, amounting to an epiphany, I was overwhelmed by a sudden and pleasing awareness that I was in union with the universe. I could reach out and touch the stars and their trillions of atoms would be the same as mine. The feeling of inclusion has never left me.

The next day, our guide told us we would die if we tried for the summit, so we chose life and headed back. There was some disappointment, but to me, there was a deeper satisfaction — that of knowing I had challenged myself and had decided my own fate. The journey was much more than summiting and conquering a mountain. The ultimate journey was within and to conquer oneself.

Chapter 12

Survivorship

The history of cancer goes back to ancient times. As a species, we have struggled to understand it, to control it, to prevent and treat it — to survive it. Ancient Egyptians blamed the gods. Hippocrates, often called the founder of modern medicine, believed that cancer was caused by an imbalance of 'black bile' in the body. He used the Greek term for crab 'karkinos' (carcinos) to describe cancer, and we see this terminology still in use today. Cancer was considered incurable. In the 1800s, when anaesthesia became available, surgery as a method for treating cancer escalated, and in the early 1900s radiation therapy emerged. These two treatment methods dominated cancer therapy until around the 1960s. Chemotherapy as a cancer treatment rapidly expanded after World War II. Hormone therapy also came into the cancer war chest in the mid-1900s, and in 1966 Charles Huggins won a Nobel Prize in Physiology or Medicine for his discoveries concerning hormonal treatment of prostatic cancer. While all these important medical developments were happening however, the perspective of the patient themselves was not a clear area of focus. This started to change in the late 1980s. The idea that the quality of life of the patient and their experience of cancer mattered became a topic of discussion.

One key event was in 1986 when the National Coalition for Cancer Survivorship (NCCS) was founded by cancer survivors in the United States to advocate for all people affected by cancer. The NCCS defined survivorship as extending from the time of diagnosis and for the balance of life; a definition then expanded to include family, friends and caregivers. It took another ten years before major health bodies, such as the National Institutes for Health National Cancer Institute, noticeably took on the idea of cancer survivorship. And while now many national and international health organisations talk about improving quality of life and the patient and family experience of cancer, they are about 70 years behind what people with cancer have been asking for and doing themselves to achieve this goal.

In a relatively recent example, the incidence of prostate cancer in Australia dramatically increased in the early 1990s as a result of the introduction of the prostate-specific antigen blood test as the first (and still only, although now more refined) way to detect prostate cancer early, when it is potentially curable. At this time, information and support services for men with prostate cancer were very hard to find, and so men themselves in a grassroots movement established community-based support groups all over the country, supporting each other and lobbying hard for improvements in services and treatments. Connected to this was the formation of the Prostate Cancer Foundation of Australia in 1996, and in time the two movements merged to become the one peak voice for men with prostate cancer and their families. For those of you who are interested in this movement an open access article describing it is included in the Appendix of this book.

Treatments for prostate cancer have, of course, dramatically changed over the past two decades. Robot-assisted surgeries, refined methods of radiation therapy, a range of different hormone-blocking treatments, new chemotherapy regimens, and targeted or personalised medicine that may be prescribed based on genomic profiling are now available in many, although not all, settings. Despite all these positive developments, research shows that men and their doctors, and the nurses and allied health professionals who look after them, report the experience of prostate cancer as being challenging, medically focused, and uncoordinated, with men's support needs often still not being adequately met. In all of this medical progress, change and evolution, the patient experience *should* be the central focus. Patient priorities and preferences *should* guide each step and each decision. Survivorship matters. So what do we need to do?

A Consensus Approach to Survivorship in Prostate Cancer

Key aspects of survivorship that both men with prostate cancer and their health care team agree about are:

- Health Promotion and Advocacy
- Shared Management
- Vigilance
- Personal Agency
- Care Coordination
- Evidence-based Survivorship Interventions.

Details of how these six domains were developed are included in the Appendix Section 4 with an open-access link. So what does this all mean?

Health Promotion and Advocacy

For men and their partners, *Health Promotion and Advocacy* means having accurate information about prostate cancer for yourself, your family and your community. This also means advocating for better treatment and services when needed. And it means taking a men's health approach to prostate cancer where all aspects of your health and wellbeing matter.

What can I do? Be informed and be active in seeking information from credible and reliable sources such as those listed in the Appendix of this book. Share what you know about prostate cancer with people who matter to you, in your family and close networks. Help raise the profile of prostate cancer, so it is a topic we can all talk about as an important men's health issue. Encourage other men to be proactive about their health and understand about their prostate cancer risk. Perhaps connect with local support groups in your area and see how you might help. Support the Prostate Cancer Foundation of Australia in its work to improve this area of men's health. Be informed. Add your voice to the community conversation about prostate cancer. Be heard.

Shared Management

This means being an equal partner in your health care, sharing decision-making with your health care team and sharing how you will tackle challenges as they arise. Being an equal partner starts at the beginning with informed decision-making around testing and treatment, under-

Prostate Cancer Survivorship Essentials

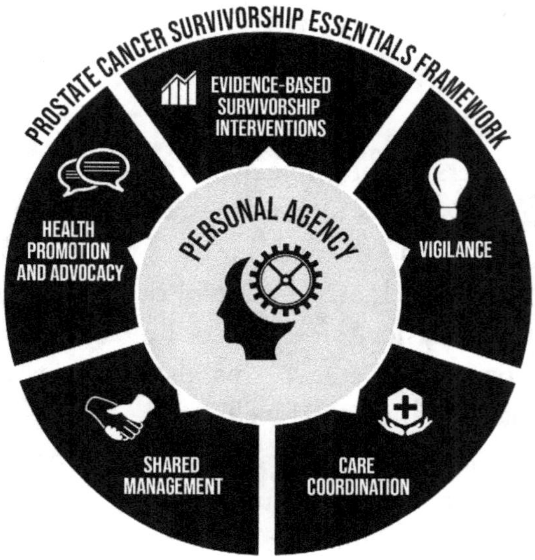

[Adapted from Dunn J, Green A, Ralph N, Newton R, Kneebone A, Frydenberg M, Chambers SK. Prostate Cancer Survivorship Essentials Framework: Guidelines for Practitioners (2020). British Journal of Urology International. https://doi.org/10.1111/bju.15159.]

standing and managing the physical and psychosocial effects of treatment and of the disease at every stage of the disease.

What can I do? Be clear with your health care team about how involved you want to be in decisions about your care, and who else you want to be involved, such as your partner or other family members or supports. Question lists can help guide the conversation with your doctor, nurse or other health professional and are a great memory guide. Plan in advance of your consultation with your doctor and work out what questions you need answered, perhaps with the support of a partner or a close friend.

Being informed will help you be more action-oriented in how you work with the team. Make sure your family doctor is also connected into the team so that they are well prepared to support you.

Vigilance

Vigilance refers to the clinical surveillance of patients from health professionals across the survivorship experience from diagnosis and through life, and this includes not only physical issues such as the control of the cancer and management of physical side effects but also other illnesses that can occur as we age. This also includes checking on your emotional and social wellbeing.

What can I do? Communicate your concerns and how you are going both physically and emotionally to your health care team. They might not always pick up on your concerns and they can't read your mind. Don't assume the effects or issues you are concerned about are not important or that your doctor or nurse is not interested or too busy to help. If it matters to you, then it matters to your health care team. How do you think you are going? There are tools around to help gauge your level of stress. For example, there is a 'Distress Thermometer' that has a symptom checklist with it, and a link to this is in the Appendix. Your doctor or nurses may have already asked you this question: How distressed have you felt over the past week on a scale of 0 – no distress, to 10 – extreme distress? If you are 4 or over on this scale, then your doctor or nurse needs to know so they can work with you on what support you might need. Check the items on the checklist to get a sense of what might be most strongly influencing how you are feeling.

Ask your doctor for a survivorship care plan that details your treatments and follow up checks. Survivorship care plans typically include a treatment summary, a plan about surveillance and follow up tests, and possible treatment side effects that might occur. Lifestyle tips and wellbeing pointers are also often included. Your doctor may have already provided you with a plan, and if not look at the links in the Appendix about Survivorship for examples you can download. Ask your doctor or nurse to complete this with you at your next visit. Involve your partner or family, so you are all across the plan.

Personal Agency

Personal agency belongs to you. This is your ability to be self-aware in how you are going and what you need, to seek assistance when you need it, and to manage your own health where you can. This does not mean going it alone. It means finding out who is there to help, what you can do yourself and what others can offer, and being an active part of the team.

What can I do? A good first step is to set survivorship goals that most matter to you. In thinking of the months and years ahead, what are the health and wellbeing or survivorship goals that you would like to work towards? These might be goals around physical activity or mental wellbeing; you may also have goals around urinary control or other physical symptoms. Strengthening your intimate relationship or perhaps looking to develop one might be on your list. Once you have your goals clear, then identify the information and other support you might need to achieve these goals. Set targets that are achievable and put an action plan in place with a timeline. Be prepared to be flexible and problem solve as you go along. This approach will help you to feel more in control of your care and the plan going forward.

Care Coordination

Care Coordination is about your health care team working together to get you the best care possible in a 'right place at the right time' approach. It means the team of different types of doctors, nurses and allied health who are looking after you are working together and communicating effectively.

What can I do? Ask your doctor or prostate cancer specialist nurse who is the lead person coordinating your care to give you a list of all the people who are in your health care team, what their job is, and how you can contact them if you need to. Also, ask who is keeping your family doctor in the loop. If you move to a different treatment approach you might need to ask these questions again.

Evidence-based Survivorship Interventions

Your time and energy are valuable. Being evidence-based is about directing your time, energy and resources to strategies that have strong evidence to support their effectiveness. Good evidence is available for the effectiveness of a range of emotional and mental wellbeing approaches, and this book includes many of these evidence-based strategies. As discussed earlier, there is excellent evidence for the benefits of exercise medicine. And for overall wellness, good nutritional habits are important. Sexual health support tailored to individual men in different age groups and with different sexual orientations and partner relationships is also an area where good evidence exists about what works, and the evidence here continues to grow.

What can I do? The tip here is to be discerning about the strategies you use to achieve your survivorship goals. When you consult practitioners, either personally or by sourcing self-help programs, check the evidence they have to back up their claims of how this might help you. If you are unsure about this contact a reputable cancer organisation such as those listed in the Appendix of this book and ask for advice. There will be different ways to get this type of support, and this could include face-to-face services, telehealth, web-based programs or self-help guides. Talk to other men who have had prostate cancer to see what they have found helpful and accessible. Tap into this valuable resource of personal experience.

Conclusion

The road ahead is yours to travel. Parts of the future may seem clear — some of it will be uncertain — either way, it belongs to you. We can't always choose what comes our way. But we can choose how we respond and find our own best solutions. Reach out, connect. Truly you are not alone.

Appendix

This is a brief list of places to you might look to for more detailed information on specific issues. For medical or treatment questions your doctor is the best first point of call for advice that is personalised to your situation. Contact details were accurate at time of printing.

1. Helpful Information

Facing Prostate Cancer

The Prostate Playbook: Keep It. Healthy. Craig Allingham. Redsok Publications, Australia. 2019. ISBN 978098706670.

Gay and Bisexual Men Living with Prostate Cancer From Diagnosis to Recovery. Edited by Jane Ussher, Janette Perz, and B. R. Simon Rosser. Harrington Park Press, LLC.

Sex and Sexuality

Saving Your Sex Life: A Guide for Men with Prostate Cancer. John P. Mulhall. Hilton Publishing, Bethesda, MD. 2010. ISBN 9780980064964. Also available as an ebook on Kindle.

After Prostate Cancer: A What-comes-next guide to a safe and informed recovery. Arnold Melman MD and Rosemary E. Newnham. Oxford University Press, New York. 2011. ISBN 9780195399660. Also available as an ebook on Kindle.

A gay man's guide to prostate cancer. Gerald Perlman and Jack Drescher. Haworth Medical Press, United States. 2005. ISBN 9781560235521.

www.renewintimacy.org The *Center for Intimacy after Cancer Therapy, Inc.* is a non-profit organisation dedicated to helping couples renew their intimacy after cancer. Founders and Co-Executive Directors: Ralph and Barbara Alterowitz.

Urinary Problems

Conquering Incontinence: A New and Physical Approach to a Freer Lifestyle Exercise. Peter Dornan. Allen & Unwin, Australia 2003. ISBN 9781741141443. Also available as an ebook on Kindle.

Prostate Recovery MAP: Men's Action Plan. Craig Allingham. Redsok, Australia. 2013. ISBN 9780987076656.

Mindfulness and Meditation

Happy For No Good Reason: A meditators guide. Swami Shankarananda. Motilal Banasidass, India. 2004. ISBN 9788120820050. Also available as an ebook on Kindle.

Full Catastrophe Living (Revised Edition): Using the Wisdom of Your Body and Mind to Face Stress, Pain, and Illness. Jon Kabat-Zinn. Delta Publishing, United Kingdom. 2013. ISBN 9780345536938. Also available as an ebook on Kindle.

Complementary Medicine

Promoting Wellness for Prostate Cancer Patients: A guide for men and their families. Fourth Edition. Mark A Moyad. Spry Publishing LLC, United States. 2013. ISBN 9781938170034.

Wellbeing

What Women (and Their Men) Need to Know About Prostate Cancer. Irena Madjar in collaboration with Gail Tingle. Prostate Survival Alliance Inc., Australia. 2008. ISBN 9780646482965.

2. Advice about Exercise

www.essa.org.au Exercise and Sports Science Australia (ESSA) — provide details of registered exercise professionals with University qualifications who are able to conduct exercise training with people who have had cancer or other chronic illnesses. The ESSA website has a section in their main page on How to Find an Accredited Exercise Physiologist (AEP) and you can select 'cancer' as a speciality: https://www.essa.org.au/find-aep.

www.acsm.org American College of Sports Medicine (ACSM) provides a similar service.

www.bases.org.uk The British Association of Sport and Exercise Sciences, BASES provides a similar service in the United Kingdom.

3. Sources of Information and Support

Australia

www.pcfa.org.au/support To contact a prostate cancer support group in your local area look up the *Prostate Cancer Foundation of Australia* website or call freecall: 1800 220 099. The Prostate Cancer Foundation of Australia (PCFA) is a broad-based community organisation and the peak national body for prostate cancer in Australia dedicated to reducing the impact of prostate cancer on Australian men, their partners, families and the wider community. PCFA can provide you with written information about prostate cancer and its treatment and can connect you to relevant services.

The *Cancer Council Helpline* is a free, confidential telephone information and support service run by Cancer Councils in each state and territory in Australia. Specially trained staff are available to answer questions about cancer and provide support. Call 13 11 20 (local call cost from anywhere in Australia but mobile calls charged at mobile rates), open between 9am and 5pm, Monday to Friday, however some states have extended hours.

New Zealand

www.prostate.org.nz/support-groups To contact a prostate cancer support group in your local area look up the *Prostate Cancer Foundation of New Zealand* website or call 0800 477 678. The Prostate Cancer Foundation of New Zealand aims to help those recently diagnosed with prostate cancer, and survivors of prostate cancer, to lead productive and full lives through shared counselling and discussions.

www.cancernz.org.nz The *Cancer Society of New Zealand* has a free Cancer Information Helpline, 0800 CANCER (226 237), which supplies booklets, information sheets and other information resources which can also be downloaded directly from their website.

North America

www.ustoo.org *Us TOO International Prostate Cancer Education and Support Network* is a non-profit, grassroots organisation that provides support for prostate cancer patients, survivors, their spouses and partners and families. More details can be found on their website. They have a toll free line to link for patients and concerned others to resources regarding diagnosis, treatment options and support systems and phone support from a prostate cancer survivor. Call 1-800-80-UsTOO (1-800-808-7866), open between 9am and 5pm, Monday to Friday, Central Time.

http://malecare.org *Malecare* develops practical, life-enhancing men's health programs and has a focus on gay and bisexual men's survivorship. Malecare runs a series of workshops and Prostate Cancer Support groups throughout the United States in areas of newly diagnosed cancer support groups, advanced prostate cancer, men diagnosed under age 50 and gay cancer survivor support.

Canada

www.prostatecancer.ca In early 2020, *Prostate Cancer Canada* amalgamated with the *Canadian Cancer Society*. As well as connecting you to support groups the website also hosts a series of Expert Angle webinars, which cover many different prostate cancer related topics.

United Kingdom

www.tackleprostate.org The *National Federation of Prostate Cancer Support Groups* can connect you to a support group through their free Helpline on 0800 035 5302 or via their website.

https://prostatecanceruk.org *Prostate Cancer UK* provides a free hotline and live website chat run by specialist nurses, which can be accessed via their website or by calling 0800 074 8383. There are also options for local and online support groups, a dedicated online community, and one-to-one support provided by trained volunteers.

www.prostatescotland.org.uk *Prostate Scotland* is a Scottish charity set up to provide information, advice and help on prostate cancer. They can connect you to support groups across the country. They also provide a range of information.

Europe

www.europa-uomo.org *Europa Uomo* (Italian for Europe man) is a European advocacy movement representing 27 prostate patients' groups in countries across Europe. Details of member organisations in each country, and in the countries' language, can be found on their website.

4. Survivorship

Dunn J, Casey C, Sandoe D, Hyde MK, Cheron-Sauer M-C, Lowe A, Oliffe J & Chambers SK. *Advocacy, Support and Survivorship in Prostate Cancer.* (2018) *European Journal of Cancer Care. 27(2)* e12644. doi: 10.1111/ecc.12644 — This article describes the development of the prostate cancer support network in Australia. Direct open access link: **https://onlinelibrary.wiley.com/doi/full/10.1111/ecc.12644**

Dunn J, Green A, Ralph N, Newton R, Kneebone A, Frydenberg M, Chambers SK. Prostate Cancer Survivorship Essentials Framework: Guidelines for Practitioners (2020). British Journal of Urology International. https://doi.org/10.1111/bju.15159. — This paper further describes the framework for prostate cancer survivorship from Chapter 12 and was developed by clinical and community groups in Australia and New Zealand. Direct

open access link:
https://bjuijournals.onlinelibrary.wiley.com/doi/10.1111/bju.15159

www.cancer.net/survivorship/follow-care-after-cancer treatment/asco-cancer-treatment-and-survivorship-care-plans The *American Society of Clinical Oncology* has developed two forms to help people diagnosed with cancer keep track of the treatment they received and medical care they may need in the future: a Cancer Treatment Plan and a Survivorship Care Plan.

www.petermac.org/sites/default/files/media-uploads/ACSC_Factsheet_SurvivorshipCarePlans.pdf This is an Australian version developed by the *Australian Cancer Survivorship Centre.*

www.prostate.org.au/awareness/for-healthcare-professionals/screening-for-distress The Prostate Cancer Foundation of Australia has a *Distress Screening Tool* for health professionals to use with men to assess their level of distress and identify key problems. The tool is to help your health care provider ensure that your emotional and psychological wellbeing needs are being addressed. A score of 4 or more on the Distress Thermometer needs a conversation with your doctor or nurse about how you are tracking.

www.servicesaustralia.gov.au/individuals/services/centrelink/disability-support-pension/what-resources-are-available/dis-ability-employment-services/work-assist Work Assist is an Australian government service that can help to redesign your job so you can keep working, change your workplace so you can continue to work, or get specialised equipment to help you do your job.

5. Other Useful Websites

www.prostatenet.com *The Prostate Net* is an international organisation that uses a matrix of informational techniques (web site, 800#, email and personal team counsellors, public forums, newsletters and community disease interventions) to address disease risk awareness and early disease detection.

Notes and Reflections

Notes and Reflections

Notes

Notes

Notes

Notes

www.ingramcontent.com/pod-product-compliance
Lightning Source LLC
LaVergne TN
LVHW080021210926
848481LV00011B/3078
* 9 7 8 1 9 2 5 6 4 4 5 5 5 *